Get Off The
PMS & Perimenopausal
Roller Coaster

*Learn 9 Natural Fast Track Solutions
to Balanced Hormones*

Brenda Eastwood, RNCP

Maximum Results Inc.
Victoria, British Columbia, Canada

***Get Off the PMS and Perimenopausal Roller Coaster,
Learn 9 Natural Fast Track Solutions to Balanced Hormones***

Copyright © 2013 Brenda Eastwood.
All rights reserved.

Library and Archives Canada Cataloguing in Publication

Eastwood, Brenda, 1958-
      Get off the PMS & perimenopausal roller coaster : learn 9
      fast track solutions to balanced hormones / Brenda Eastwood.

ISBN 978-0-9918818-0-2

      1. Premenstrual syndrome–Alternative treatment–Popular works.
      2. Perimenopause–Alternative treatment–Popular works. I. Title.
      RG165.E28 2013   618.1'72   C2013-901331-8

Printed in Canada

Publisher: Maximum Results Inc.
For information contact maximumresults@shaw.ca

Cover Design and Illustrations by Chris Price
Formatting by Diane Mendez

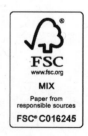

FSC
www.fsc.org
MIX
Paper from
responsible sources
FSC® C016245

Table of Contents

LIFESTYLE STRATEGIES FOR A LIFETIME

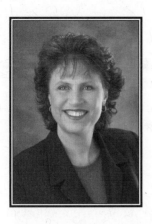

About the Author
Brenda Eastwood

Brenda Eastwood is passionate about helping other women. "When I was heading into menopause at the early age of 32, I had no idea what was happening to me and what I could do about it. I suffered with flooding, long or irregular periods, insomnia, hot flashes, night sweats, weight gain, mood swings and severe fatigue. Because I was going through perimenopause prematurely, nothing I had learned was working for me, and none of the professionals I sought out were able to help. But through research, education, experimentation, and perseverance I was able to discover natural solutions to all of my hormonal health challenges. Now, I would like all women to learn what I know so they can feel as good as I do."

After 17 years of running a very successful private practice, Brenda decided she wanted to make a bigger contribution to improving women's health. Since 1999 she has been sharing her knowledge through workshops, seminars, audio programs, TV, radio, teleclasses and her unique on-line support program called the Inner Circle. You know you are in capable hands as she draws on more than 30 years of experience as a Registered Nutritional Consulting Practitioner, working with women all over the globe.

Brenda's seminars are far from ordinary. She is a knowledgeable, gifted, high-energy speaker who has her audiences shaking with laughter as she discusses subjects that aren't normally discussed in a fun, yet totally professional manner.

Brenda is not your typical nutritionist. She is a realist who believes in minimal input for maximum results. Having overcome her own health challenges, she has a deep sensitivity to women's health concerns and understands the challenges that women face.

She takes all the guesswork out of "how to achieve hormonal balance and optimal health." She has helped turn around the lives of thousands of women by providing them with step-by-step strategies that are affordable, easy to incorporate and produce outstanding and long-lasting results.

If you are tired of confusing, contradictory opinions, and complicated health regimes, you will find Brenda's practical and simple approach to be a breath of fresh air. Not only does she make sense, her techniques actually work!

Acknowledgements

Now I know why I procrastinated for so long on publishing a book. It is a massive undertaking. I would never have taken it on if it were not for all the clients who told me how much a book like this was needed and the constant encouragement and endless support I received from my friends and family.

My husband, Adrian Eastwood, is my rock. He continually lifts the burden of day-to-day concerns for me so that I can stay focused on all my end goals, including this book. He is a never-ending source of strength and comfort to me. I can't imagine my life without him. There are no words to express my appreciation and gratitude. I love you.

Megan Bocsik has been so much more than my nutritional partner. When I asked her to do the first round of editing on my manuscript draft, I was more than pleasantly surprised – I was truly AMAZED. She put her heart and soul into the edits as if it was her own book and did a brilliant job. Her insights and suggestions have made a huge difference to the success of the finished copy. Massive kudos to you Megan, I can't thank you enough. I look forward to a long and fabulous relationship with you.

Christine Awram, dear friend and founder of Woman of Worth WOW Events, has been the proverbial dog on my pant leg that I couldn't shake loose. Ever since I met Christine she has continually prodded me to write a book. Her final "love shove" was inviting me to *An Evening for Women of Worth* with Julie Salisbury, Founder of Influence Publishing. Apparently that was the last piece of inspiration and motivation that I needed. Thank you, Christine, for your never-ending faith in my abilities and for never letting go of my pant leg!

Michael Losier, author of *Law of Attraction* and *Law of Connection*, has been an incredible mentor and friend. True to his word, when I was ready to write this book, he was there to share his experience and guidance. It was through a creative brainstorming session with him that the title and layout of the book took shape. I am so grateful for "attracting" him into my life.

Any new author needs a friend like Jan Janzen. Oh my goodness, if it were not for her, I would truly never have gotten through this process. She is the successful author of four books including *Breast Health Exposed, 21 Secrets Most Doctors Will Never Tell You About Your Breasts*. She shared with me all of the ins and outs, who to contact, what to do, what not to do, and most importantly gave me information I didn't know I would even need to know. Your friendship and your continual help mean more to me than you will ever know!

Many years ago I got the notion to work with Linda Adams on a book. Even though it took some 20 years to come about, I can tell you it was a wise idea. Linda was my second-in-line editor, who brought humor to the tedious job of rewrites. Her tireless devotion to my book and her recommendations were always spot on. Thank you from the bottom of my heart.

My cousin, Jaymie Hackman, gave me valuable insights on changes that would make the book easier to read and comprehend. Thank you Jaymie for your contribution and support. You have no idea how much it means to me.

Chris Price, the illustrator, was able to make this part of the journey a pleasure rather than a chore. I appreciate his patience with my questions. He always seemed to know exactly what I wanted. From professional charts to fun cartoons, his work truly completes this book.

Carla Higgins was another incredible person who showed up to help proof the manuscript. Her attention to detail, and many insights proved to be a huge blessing. Thank you so much Carla!

Diane Mendez, my final editor and formatter, has so much experience and expertise with publishing books that I felt totally at ease with the formatting process. Thank you Diane for making this book such an easy read.

Last but certainly not least, is Karen Laharty. She is a friend of Megan's who volunteered to read the material and give feedback from a lay person's perspective. Unbeknownst to me, she had been an editor in a previous job. Those skills certainly shone through. Thank you, Karen, for the generosity of your time and remarkable talent.

Introduction

Whether this is your first or your twentieth attempt at resolving your hormonal issues, I guarantee it will be your last.

My nine Natural Fast Track Solutions have a proven record that you can trust. Thousands of women just like you are now symptom-free and in control of their bodies.

In your search for a solution, you have likely heard these promises before. Advertisements make it sound like all you need is this new miracle formulation and *voila* your hormonal troubles will disappear. But the only thing that disappeared was more of your valuable time and money. Even though you were disappointed, you tried again.

You likely visited a health food store, treated yourself to the spa, tried a new diet, searched the Internet or went to the library. But for all your efforts, you didn't notice much of a change. You are still suffering.

You may have been tempted to give up or you are simply wondering "What is wrong with me? Why isn't anything working?"

Let me assure you. There is nothing wrong with you.

The reason you have experienced little to no results, or the results you have achieved haven't lasted, is that you are unique. Hormonal issues develop for different reasons; inherited tendencies, lifestyles, diets, stress levels and nutritional requirements. How can there possibly be a one-size-fits-all hormone balancing product or program?

You can't give Miranda, whose hormones are out of whack from a Candida overgrowth, the same products or protocol as you give Julie, whose hormones are out of sync because she has severe adrenal fatigue.

That is why this book is different.

As a women's health specialist with over 30 years of real life experience, helping women just like you resolve their hormonal health challenges, I have discovered what works and what doesn't.

I have mapped out a step-by-step protocol so you can discover the underlying causes of your hormone imbalance. Then I give you detailed instructions on how to create and follow your own unique road map to balanced hormones.

I have either been where you are today or have been through a similar experience with a client; and I guarantee that if you are willing to follow my step-by-step system, you can create not only the results you want, but those you so deserve.

Yours in Total Health,

Brenda

CHAPTER 1

Getting Started

Conventional Medicine VS Alternative Medicine

The practice of conventional medicine has its greatest strength and value in the hospital emergency room. Acute crisis intervention demands state-of-the-art, life-saving drugs and surgery. There is NO alternative to medical treatment for most of life's major traumas.

Conventional medicine is the clear choice when it comes to the treatment of broken bones, lacerations, severed tendons, heart attacks and organ failures.

On the other hand, conventional medicine leaves a lot to be desired when it comes to the treatment or prevention of chronic illnesses like arthritis, cancer, diabetes and heart disease. It has no safe treatment for everyday health concerns such as migraines, hot flashes, depression, fatigue and more. It certainly offers very limited hope to women suffering with PMS (premenstrual syndrome) and perimenopausal symptoms, as you may have already discovered.

Unfortunately, misinformation and lack of education stand in the way of the majority of people benefiting from alternative medicine. Rationality, common sense and scientific proof have been bypassed in order to protect the financial interests of the pharmaceutical and medical industries.

With that awareness, I ask that you try to keep an open mind. There will likely be many times that my material will contradict everything you have ever heard or have been programmed to believe.

The majority of medical doctors receive only a few hours of nutrition education. Just as you would not ask a plumber for accounting advice, it doesn't make sense to go to your doctor for education or advice on nutrition.

What does make sense is to seek out an expert regarding your problem or concern. You have made the right choice seeking out my advice for a natural way to balance your hormones.

The goal of this book is to help you get the results you want as quickly as possible with the least amount of cost and effort.

Remember, it took time to get where you are now, so it will take time to recover and rejuvenate. Thankfully your body is forgiving, and with the right raw materials to work with, it can repair itself in much less time than it took to get where you are today. Think progress, not perfection.

The suggested nutritional strategies I provide will move you closer to your goals, but it is important to take action at a rate that is comfortable for you. It doesn't matter how much or how little you tackle and at what pace, I just encourage you to take affirmative steps daily. You can't simply read this book and hope your symptoms will get better via osmosis. To get results you must take action.

I know you are looking forward to having boundless energy, a slim body, great moods and more, so let's get going!

CHAPTER 2

How the Book Is Organized

What I have learned and could teach you would fill dozens of books. As you go through this book, remember that it can't cover everything I know, but it does cover everything <u>you need to know</u> about balancing your hormones.

You might be quite surprised to discover what I *do* and *don't* discuss. For example, I will talk to you about the importance of proper bowel function, but I won't talk to you about exercise.

I have selected only the <u>most</u> critical steps for you to take to achieve <u>fast, safe and effective results</u>.

About Chapter 3: Do We Really Need Vitamins?

You may be tempted to jump into the book at a place that grabs your attention the most, but please start with Chapter 3: **Do We Really Need Vitamins?**

This chapter explains why I believe you must take supplements if you want balanced hormones and optimal health.

Even though supplements are critical to your success, you can't rely on supplements alone. Supplements should be just that, a "supplement" to your everyday diet.

The definition of the word *supplement* is: something added to complete a thing, supply a deficiency, or reinforce or extend a whole.

Diet and lifestyle are also exceptionally important, and that is why I have dedicated eight chapters to the topic. If you <u>only</u> want to utilize these lifestyle strategies to positively impact your hormones, then you have the option to go directly to **Lifestyle Strategies for a Lifetime,** found in chapters 15 to 22.

I have chosen to start with supplements and address lifestyle strategies later, because I have learned that:

1. Women are so darn busy. If I give them a program that is hard to do, they won't stick with it. Taking vitamins may seem like an easier place to start than with bigger lifestyle changes.

2. Mass media has brainwashed women to believe everything happens quickly, and I know this is what you expect. By recommending concentrated nutrients as your first step, I am giving you tools to provide your body with the best opportunity to make its swiftest recovery. If I started you with lifestyle strategies or didn't recommend supplements at all, the results would be so slow in arriving that you would probably give up on balancing your hormones. Then you'd be right back where you started, frustrated, with hormonal symptoms that are disrupting your full enjoyment of life.

3. When women see positive results, they are encouraged to stick with their program. I learned this lesson in the early days of running my private practice. For example, when women would come to me for weight loss, I would first give them supplements to help them eliminate their fatigue. Once they had more energy, they were able to do a bit of exercise and make nutritious meals. That would then start the weight loss process, making it easier to say no to the chocolate cake, and so forth. From there, we were on a positive roll.

About Chapter 4: Hormones 101

This chapter is crucial to your success.

I don't expect you to become a hormone specialist, but you do need to comprehend the basics of what is happening in your body so you understand how to balance your hormones. It is far easier to make a change or take a supplement if you understand WHY you are doing it as opposed to just doing it because you were told to.

I have taken enormous amounts of technical information and made it easy to understand. This knowledge will not only help you to eliminate your current hormonal symptoms, but it will serve you well into the future as your body changes. With this know-how, you will always be able to make more informed decisions regarding your health.

Knowledge is Power

About Chapter 5: The First Step – The Fast Track Foundation Overview

There are three initial steps that are the same for each woman, so I have termed this set of steps accordingly as the **Fast Track Foundation**.

To really make the **Fast Track Foundation** FAST, I start with an overview so you can take immediate action.

If you only experience mild PMS (premenstrual syndrome) or perimenopausal symptoms, the **Fast Track Foundation** may be all you need to eliminate your hormonal symptoms.

If you have moderate to severe PMS or perimenopausal symptoms, the **Fast Track Foundation** will give you some immediate relief; but to completely restore hormonal balance, you will also need to address other underlying factors.

No matter how great your results are with the **Fast Track Foundation**, I encourage you to explore the other factors that can influence your hormones, as these could become issues at a later date.

For example, let's say that by the time you come to the section on adrenal fatigue, your hormone symptoms have disappeared and you don't feel the need to read any further. I encourage you to carry on because it could be that you have the beginning stages of adrenal fatigue that haven't yet affected your hormones but are starting to cause other symptoms such as hay fever or joint pain. By working through the entire book, you will be going beyond balancing your hormones, and you will be headed for the ultimate goal: optimal health.

The ultimate goal:
Optimal Health

THE 9 NATURAL FAST TRACK SOLUTIONS

About Chapters 6 to 8

These chapters go into more detail about the **Fast Track Foundation**.

About Chapters 9 to 14

These chapters will guide you through the other factors that could be influencing your hormone balance and/or your health. They are mapped out in the order you should approach them in your hormone balancing program.

If you want to feel happy, energized and slim, in the least amount of time, then follow the protocol I have set out for you in these chapters. Choosing the place you would like to start, as opposed to choosing the place you should start, will not only delay your results, it will likely cause you to waste precious time, energy and money.

When To Break Protocol

If you are contemplating a hysterectomy because you have a fibroid or are bleeding excessively at each period, there is no time to read through this book and proceed one by one through the underlying issues.

Although you will need to work through each chapter in due course, my experience has been that women in dire straits need to take a shortcut, and fast. Therefore, if you would like to give yourself the opportunity to bypass the hysterectomy, I strongly suggest that you begin immediately with the **Fast Track Foundation** and go directly to Chapter 12: **Fast Track Solution Seven - Reversing An Iodine Deficiency** and Chapter 14: **Fast Track Solution Nine - The Appropriate Use of Natural Bio-Identical Progesterone Cream**.

LIFESTYLE STRATEGIES FOR A LIFETIME

About Chapters 15 to 22

Though these chapters are placed last, they are still exceptionally important. In fact, there will be several times as you work through the Fast Track Solutions that I recommend putting a book mark in your spot and jumping ahead to this section so that you can learn some lifestyle strategies to speed up your results.

Undoubtedly, some strategies will be hard for you, while others will be easy. You may already be doing some of them, so there will be nothing to change. But you might find another strategy quite difficult to adjust to. When I am asking you to do things in a different way than you are accustomed to, such as changing a particular way of eating, it can be very difficult, as it means breaking those old habits and establishing new and better ones. Think beyond the difficulty of these moments and remember to begin with the end in mind.

You will need to make a commitment to these lifestyle changes and they do require a concerted effort. If you get frustrated or overwhelmed and feel like quitting, don't! When you feel like giving up, remember why it is you started and stick it out. The rewards will be worth it.

The important thing to remember is that all positive changes are taking you one step closer to your goals. When it comes to your health, it is better to take consistent baby steps rather than sporadic giant leaps.

I have seen woman after woman make too many New Year's resolutions, which makes them unrealistic to keep. You know the ones – *I am going to exercise daily, spend more time with my family, cut back at work, learn a new language, quit smoking and lose 30 lbs.* These are just too many resolutions to tackle all at one time. The women, who make too many resolutions, usually find themselves making the same ones year after year.

I am not saying this to give you an excuse for not making necessary lifestyle changes, but rather to make two simple points:

1. The **Lifestyle Strategies For a Lifetime** are critical to your health and hormones, no matter what life stage you are in.

2. You need to make a realistic plan of action in order to successfully accomplish these strategies.

When you feel like quitting, think about why you started

About Chapter 23: Extra Support For Painful Menstrual Cramps

This title is self-explanatory.

LOTS OF ADDITIONAL SUPPORT

You will notice that all the way through this book, I reference other authors or websites that will offer you additional support.

I also refer you to my website www.HormoneRollerCoaster.com, where you will find:

1. Free worksheets to print.

2. Free articles and reports to further your education on achieving optimal health and hormone balance.

3. A subscription to my complimentary monthly newsletter, which provides leading-edge health discoveries, along with valuable hormone balancing tips, notifications of radio interviews and opportunities to attend my seminars, workshops, teleclasses or webinars.

"When health is absent,
wisdom cannot reveal itself,
art cannot manifest,
strength cannot fight,
wealth becomes useless, and
intelligence cannot be applied."

~Herophilus

CHAPTER 3

Do We Really Need Vitamins?

I believe it is absolutely essential to take daily nutritional supplements. These should be:

- superior quality
- properly combined
- highly absorbable
- correct dosages

Here's why.

Your Body is Like a Bank Account

Let's look first at how a bank account works. You put money in, you take money out; and if you take out more than you put in, you go into overdraft and are charged penalties. If you put in more than you take out, you earn some interest. Okay, so nowadays the interest is not anything to get excited about, but nonetheless your bank account grows when you put in more than you take out.

Now think about your body as a bank account. You put nutrients in, you expend those nutrients, and if you expend more than you put in, you go into nutrient overdraft (deficiency) and your penalty is some form of health symptom(s). But if you put in more nutrients than you expend, then you have the potential to earn great health, energy and vitality.

There Are No Zero Foods

Let's look at different forms of food, starting with junk food. Most people realize it isn't nourishing them, but what they don't know is that there are no zero foods.

A food is either giving you nutrients or it is depleting your limited supply. That's right. I said <u>depleting</u> your supply.

All processed foods containing white flour, sugar, chemical additives, unhealthy fats or artificial sweeteners take nutrients directly out of your nutrient bank account. You also withdraw more nutrients every time you drink pop, alcohol or coffee, take any type of drug (legal or illegal, prescription or over-the-counter), ingest pesticides, herbicides and antibiotics, or experience stress.

Even exercise draws from your nutrient supply. If you're doing enough exercise to substantially deplete energy reserves, you're using additional nutrients for energy production and recovery. As a result, athletes are at an even higher risk of nutrient deficiencies.

Given how easily you can deplete your nutrient supply, you must really focus on putting in way more nutrients than you take out or you will go into nutrient overdraft (health issues).

Are You Earning Interest or Penalties?

Of course I would be oversimplifying to say that all your health issues are caused by nutrient deficiencies. We know that isn't true. Great health and hormone balance is created through more than just nutrition. Exercise, fresh air, DNA, sleep, and positive attitude influence your health too. And some issues may be better treated by a chiropractor, acupuncturist, or massage therapist (just to name a few).

Symptoms of Nutrient Overdraft

You may be surprised, however, through the course of this book, to discover how many of your symptoms are actually associated with nutritional deficiencies. The list below shows examples of symptoms and some of the possible associated nutritional deficiencies:

- Poor night vision: vitamin A
- Depression: omega 3, vitamin D, niacin, B1, pantothenic acid, B12, and magnesium
- Headaches: pantothenic acid, niacin, and magnesium
- Low energy: vitamin A, iodine, and pantothenic acid
- Anxiety: niacin and magnesium
- Sensation of sand in eye: B2
- Insomnia: niacin, calcium, magnesium and pantothenic acid
- Tendency to bruise easily: vitamin C
- Sore joints: MSM, vitamin C and pantothenic acid

If symptoms are largely a result of nutritional deficiencies and ill health evolves from ignoring those symptoms, then doesn't it make sense to do your best to prevent nutritional deficiencies?

Of course it does. Now the question is "how do you fill up your nutrient bank account?" Can you rely on food alone?

Why You Can't Get All Your Nutrients From Food

How familiar is the phrase "you can get all the nutrients you need from your food"? Where have you typically heard this from? Consider the source. In my experience, the people who repeat this phrase the most have the least education in the science of nutrition.

I don't disagree that this saying could be true. There is no doubt in my mind that in an ideal world your nutrients would come from your food. This is how Mother Nature intended things to be. With the help of the sun, the process of photosynthesis, and adequate water, plant roots extract hard-to-digest minerals from the soil and convert them into a form you can absorb. Then when you eat these fresh fruits, vegetables and whole grains, not only should they provide you with an array of vitamins, and antioxidants, they should also supply you with your necessary minerals.

But think about this; if plants keep taking the minerals out of the soil, eventually the soil becomes depleted. Organic farming utilizes composting, crop rotation, manure, and tilling under a green manure crop (a crop that is grown and then tilled into the ground a month or so before planting time) to maintain mineral rich soil to farm on.

Unfortunately, due to modern world agribusiness, this is no longer the case. Nowadays it is all about producing the most amount of food in the most efficient and economical way possible. This means non-organic farms use none of the above ethical practices. Instead, crops are grown with the cheapest fertilizers that supply nitrogen, phosphorus, and potassium. These three minerals are enough to make the plants grow, but they certainly aren't enough to enrich the soil so that the food you eat is supplying your needs.

You miss out on all the other vital minerals such as iron, zinc, copper, cobalt, iodine, manganese, chromium, selenium, vanadium, boron, tin, nickel, fluoride, bromine, silicon, plus many more.

To add insult to injury, these nutrient-deficient foods are then sprayed with pesticides, fungicides and herbicides, which spells out more nutrient loss rather than nutrient gain, because your body uses up nutrients to deal with all of these toxins.

The fruits and vegetables don't reach their full nutrient potential because they are picked before they are ripe.

And last but not least, these foods are often *irradiated before shipping. According to the Organic Consumers Association, irradiation damages molecules and digestive enzymes in food and creates free radicals, leading to the destruction of as much as 80% of the vitamins present.

(*Irradiation is the process of exposing food to radiation for the purpose of reducing the bacteria and other microorganisms that may be present on food. It does not however prevent re-contamination.)

And what about packaged and processed foods? Processed foods are produced by using manufacturing methods to transform raw ingredients into neatly packaged goods, which have a longer shelf life. This means they are stripped of all their nutrients such as fiber, antioxidants, vitamins, minerals and good fats. Those are then replaced with artificial ingredients and chemical additives such as monosodium glutamate (MSG), flavors, preservatives, hydrogenated oil, fillers, high-fructose corn syrup and artificial sweeteners. The appeal of these products is that they can be prepared quickly for immediate intake. But can we really call these 'foods' food?

This is only the tip of the iceberg. No food group has escaped unscathed. For every progressive step forward in agribusiness, we are set back an equal or greater number of steps in the amount of nutrients that are depleted in our food.

Another example is dairy products which are all pasteurized to protect us from certain disease-carrying germs and prevent the souring of milk. Pasteurization has supposedly moved us forward, but has also set us back in terms of nutrient quality. The high temperatures required to kill bacteria also kill the living enzymes in the milk, making it much harder to digest. Plus, the process of pasteurization destroys vitamin C and 20% of the iodine.

When you take into account an overview of everything that you eat, can you still buy into the phrase "you can get all the nutrients you need from your food"? When you study fact, not fiction, you see that even fresh food is nutrient deficient and could actually be considered a negative food because your body has to use up nutrients to neutralize the toxins.

To get all of your nutrients from food, you would need to live in that ideal world where you have time to raise your own crops on nutrient-rich soil, without pesticides and herbicides. The crops would not be picked until maturity and your foods would be prepared fresh daily. You could get safe unpasteurized milk from your own cow for drinking and making butter and cheese. You could harvest, mill, bake with and prepare whole grains that have not been stripped of their fiber, vitamins and minerals.

Yes, in an ideal world, it would be possible to get all the nutrients you need from your food. But you do not live in an ideal world. In the world you live in, you need daily nutritional supplements if you want to have vibrant health and hormonal balance.

CHAPTER 4

Hormones 101

O ften referred to as "chemical messengers," hormones carry information and instructions through the bloodstream from one group
of cells to another. In the human body, hormones influence almost
every cell, organ and function. They regulate our growth, development,
metabolism, tissue function, sexual function, reproduction, the way our
bodies utilize food and nutrients, stress response in both emergency
and non-emergency situations, our sleep patterns and even our moods.

Although we have over 50 hormones in our bodies, the two I want to
focus on are estrogen and progesterone.

The most prevalent forms of estrogen in the human body are estradiol,
estrone, and estriol. For sake of ease, throughout this book, I will refer
to all three forms of these estrogens as simply "estrogen."

Balanced Progesterone and Estrogen: What Should Happen

In a hormonally balanced woman, both estrogen and progesterone
levels are relatively low during the menstrual period. Immediately
following the period, estrogen levels rise quite rapidly and dramatically,
peaking at ovulation. It is this higher level of estrogen that stimulates
the production of your uterine lining (endometrium) in preparation for
conception.

Progesterone, on the other hand, stays relatively low during the first
half of the cycle and it peaks after ovulation occurs. Ovulation triggers
the release of progesterone into the body.

For the second phase of the cycle, from ovulation to the next period, progesterone should dominate over estrogen. Progesterone plays a vital role in making the endometrium receptive to implantation of a fertilized egg.

If conception occurs, progesterone levels remain high throughout the first trimester. At that point, the placenta takes over progesterone production, as a high amount of progesterone is needed throughout the pregnancy to maintain the nourishing lining.

A lack of progesterone can hinder a fertilized egg from implanting or staying implanted.

When conception does not occur, both estrogen and progesterone drop, causing the uterine lining to shed, which is the bleeding that is experienced when a woman gets her period. The entire cycle then repeats itself.

This is what your cycle should look like.

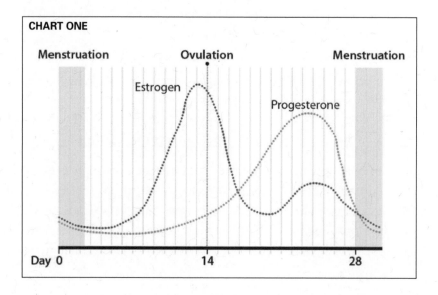

CHART ONE

Menstruation   Ovulation   Menstruation

Estrogen   Progesterone

Day 0   14   28

Estrogen Dominance: What Actually Happens

In the second half of the menstrual cycle, from ovulation to period, today's woman either doesn't produce enough progesterone OR has elevated levels of estrogen in relationship to her progesterone.

Chart one shows what your cycle should look like and chart two shows what most cycles actually look like:

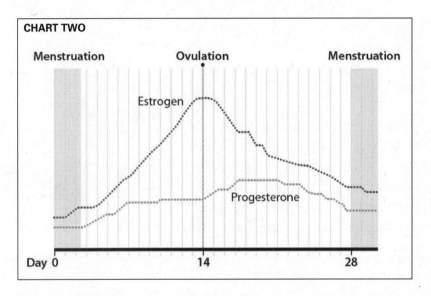

It doesn't matter which one you have, progesterone deficiency or estrogen excess, the actual discrepancy between the two (estrogen and progesterone) is referred to as "estrogen dominance." This is a term coined by Dr. John Lee, a pioneer in progesterone research and author of many books, including *What Your Doctor May Not Tell You About Perimenopause*.

It is this estrogen dominance that causes many of the hormonal issues known as PMS (premenstrual syndrome) and the unpleasant symptoms in perimenopause.

THREE LIFE STAGES

1. Menstruating Woman

This stage of life is when a woman sheds the lining of her uterus (referred to as a period) approximately every 28 days.

Most girls will get their first period around the age of 12, but it isn't uncommon to start earlier or later.

During her menstrual years, a woman can suffer with premenstrual syndrome, commonly referred to as PMS. This is a set of symptoms that may vary from one woman to another and from month to month. Symptoms can include bloating, irritability, mood swings, sore or swollen breasts, fatigue, food cravings, and more. These symptoms generally appear any time between ovulation and the first day of the period. For some women, they can last only a day or two, and in others, up to the entire two weeks leading up to their period.

Other symptoms that can be annoying or even debilitating, such as heavy flow, blood clots, nausea and cramping that come once the period starts, are not technically part of PMS, but are still part of the hormonal problem.

2. Perimenopausal Woman

Perimenopause is a new term that has evolved, and it refers to the transitional time of going from regular menstruation to menopause (no periods).

During this time, which can be as long as 10 years, the woman can get regular periods, have no periods for months, have periods every two weeks or a non-stop period for several weeks. Basically, her periods are all over the map.

On top of dealing with a completely unpredictable menstrual cycle, she can have PMS symptoms, as well as the symptoms associated with menopause such as hot flashes and night sweats.

Generally speaking, perimenopause should occur in your forties; unfortunately, in today's world, many women are going into peri-menopause in their thirties, as I did.

3. Menopausal Woman

A woman is not considered menopausal until she has gone at least 12 months in a row without a period.

The average woman can look forward to stopping her periods in her late forties or early fifties.

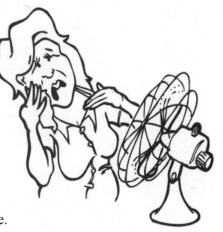

The most common symptoms of menopause are hot flashes, night sweats, and vaginal dryness. I believe the other symptoms associated with menopause are related to sleep deprivation from those night sweats as well as from the hormonal imbalances that are a carryover from the menstruating and perimenopausal stages of life.

I prefer not to use the term post-menopausal, as you are either meno-pausal or not. I think it stems from women who describe themselves as "menopausal" while having the symptoms associated with it; and when the symptoms stop, they think of themselves as "post-menopausal."

You will soon discover that you have twice as many reasons to follow through with the **Fast Track Solutions** presented here. You will not only be rewarded with freedom from your current symptoms, you will also escape the unpleasant symptoms associated with menopause.

The Same But Different

The same things that cause PMS cause perimenopausal symptoms, with only two slight differences.

1. In the perimenopausal stage, women become increasingly more estrogen dominant, which causes symptoms to worsen and/or causes the woman to experience NEW symptoms.

   The worsening of estrogen dominance is largely due to the fact that perimenopausal women don't ovulate every month. Remember, ovulation triggers the release of progesterone. So if you aren't ovulating every month then you aren't producing progesterone from your ovaries every month; and without the ovarian progesterone, you will be exceptionally estrogen dominant.

2. In the perimenopausal stage, there are times when the estrogen levels temporarily plummet and this is when those annoying menopausal symptoms show up.

Symptoms of Estrogen Dominance

#1. Proliferative Endometrium

Estrogen builds the lining of your uterus. This is necessary to prepare the uterus for an embryo to be implanted, but estrogen dominance can cause an overstimulation of this lining which can then create:

- Endometriosis (uterine lining growth outside of the uterine cavity)
- Heavy periods with or without blood clots
- Uterine fibroids
- Increased risk of endometrial cancer

This is a very common problem, especially in perimenopause. How many perimenopausal women do you know who are either currently battling an excess menstrual flow or have had a hysterectomy to stop their uncontrollable bleeding?

> *The amount of excessive bleeding*
> *is in direct correlation*
> *to the degree of estrogen dominance.*

Correct the estrogen dominance and you correct the excess flow, rectify the endometriosis and/or shrink the fibroids.

It is a known fact that if a woman with fibroids can hold onto her uterus until menopause, when there is a natural decline of her estrogen, then her fibroid(s) will shrink. This does not mean that she should simply wait until menopause. To minimize her symptoms and protect her health, a woman with fibroids should take action immediately to lower her estrogen dominance.

All doctors and medical websites will verify that estrogen dominance is responsible for fibroid growth. Here is one quote from the Cedars-Sinai patient education website: "Fibroid tumors are sensitive to changes in a woman's monthly hormone cycle. As estrogen levels tend to increase before menopause starts, many uterine fibroids start to grow. This may make the symptoms worse. After menopause, estrogen falls dramatically. This causes the fibroids to shrink (although they probably won't totally disappear) and the symptoms to diminish. If a woman is taking hormone replacement therapy (HRT), however, she will probably not experience a shrinking of the fibroids or a lessening of the symptoms."

What you won't find from these sources is the natural steps you can take to lower estrogen dominance. Without this knowledge, estrogen dominance will remain the number one cause of unnecessary hysterectomies.

#2. Breast Stimulation

In breast tissue, estrogen triggers the growth of cells that line the milk glands. This prepares the breasts to produce milk if the woman becomes pregnant. Estrogen dominance can cause too much stimulation of these cells which can result in:

- Sore, tender and/or swollen breasts
- Fibrocystic breasts
- Increased risk of breast cancer

Estrogen dominance increases your risk of breast cancer.

"Almost all risk factors associated with breast cancer are directly or indirectly related to excess estrogen, or estrogen that isn't balanced with progesterone. We believe correcting this imbalance, which Dr. Lee has termed estrogen dominance, is the essence of preventing and treating breast cancer." From the book *What Your Doctor May Not Tell You About Breast Cancer, How Hormone Balance Can Help Save Your Life.*

While there is sufficient evidence to support that estrogen dominance can increase the risk of breast cancer, there is also equal evidence to show that relying on this one component will not keep you safe from breast cancer. Through my years of counseling thousands of women, I have unquestionably witnessed a correlation between certain emotions and specific diseases such as cancer.

Although my area of expertise lies in taking care of the physical body, I definitely agree with Dr. Nelie C. Johnson, MD, who states the following: "On the subject of breast cancer, I believe it is essential to take a whole-person view. Along with physical factors, there are mental, emotional, and spiritual factors that impact our well-being. More and more medical studies and experience, including my own, are showing that diseases such as cancer, diabetes and MS are truly 'dis-eases' – the physical outcome of underlying mental and emotional stresses. As well, hormonal and nutritional balance contribute to relieving some of these stresses and provide a foundation for repair and restoring health."

For more resources on this topic I can recommend:

- Dr. Johnson's website - www.awarenessheals.ca
- Dr. Gabor Mate's book, *When the Body Says No: The Cost of Hidden Stress*

#3 Increased Body Fat

This particular body fat is commonly known as a "muffin top," "spare tire" or "middle-age spread," as it is targeted specifically around the abdomen, hips and thighs.

Here is a vicious little circle for you to think about: The more fat you have the more estrogen you will produce, and the more estrogen you produce the more fat you will store.

#4 Impaired Blood Sugar Control

Your body operates on glucose (blood sugar) just like a car operates on gasoline. You have to have it in order to keep it running. If someone extracted all the glucose from your body, you would go into a coma and be dead within minutes. The brain and central nervous system derive their support from adequate supplies of blood sugar. Therefore, low levels of blood sugar cause alterations in body and brain function.

Given your brain has to have glucose (sugar), your body has been designed to go to great lengths to protect a normal range of glucose within your blood. There is an ideal range, and your body can tolerate some fluctuation of that ideal amount. But when it gets much higher than the high end of the range and stays there, that is recognized as diabetes. When your blood sugar levels get lower than the bottom end, this is low blood sugar or hypoglycemia.

Estrogen dominance leads to or worsens already existing low blood sugar issues also known as hypoglycemia. This is why women who are already prone to minor blood sugar imbalances feel much worse during the two weeks preceding their period.

There are numerous symptoms associated with low blood sugar, but the ones you would most likely relate to during PMS are:

- Cravings for carbohydrates or sweets
- Lack of concentration
- Fatigue (especially midafternoon)
- Irritability
- Moodiness
- Depression
- Headaches
- Insomnia

Other symptoms relating to low blood sugar are:

- Nervousness
- Feelings of fear or anxiety
- Faintness, dizziness, tremors and cold sweats
- Drowsiness
- Forgetfulness, confusion
- Constant worrying, unprovoked anxiety
- Heart palpitations or rapid pulse
- Indecisiveness
- Lack of coordination
- Muscle twitching and jerking
- Sighing and yawning
- Internal trembling
- Numbness
- Crying spells

- Blurred vision
- Itching and crawling skin sensations
- Outbursts of temper
- Sleepiness
- Nightmares

#5 Subclinical Hypothyroidism

Thyroid binding globulin (TBG) is a protein responsible for carrying thyroid hormones in the bloodstream. When estrogen levels are high, the TBG will bind more thyroid hormone, decreasing the free hormone available in the blood, which can lead to subclinical hypothyroidism.

This is why women in perimenopause, who are more estrogen dominant than they will ever be at any other time in their lives, will typically start to experience symptoms of subclinical hypothyroidism. This thyroid issue, of course, follows them into menopause.

I am using the term subclinical because the medical definition differs from the nutritional definition; and sometimes your body has symptoms of hypothyroidism (low-functioning thyroid), but the blood tests do not confirm this condition.

Common symptoms of subclinical hypothyroidism are:
- Unjustified weight gain and/or difficulty losing weight
- Fatigue
- Depression
- Constipation
- Heavier, more frequent and more painful periods
- Hair loss
- Muscle cramps and joint pain
- Water retention

#6 Short Menstrual Cycles and Infertility Issues

A menstrual cycle is the time frame between the first day of your period and the first day of your next period. A normal cycle is about 26-30 days. I consider anything less than 26 days a short cycle.

One of the functions of progesterone is to hold onto your uterine lining. In the second half of your cycle, from ovulation to your period, you are supposed to produce about 20 mg of progesterone daily. If you conceive, your progesterone levels continue to rise to about 400 mg per day during the first trimester. This ensures success of the pregnancy.

If progesterone levels are too low (still called estrogen dominance), there may not be enough to hold onto the uterine lining for very long. This would cause you to have a short cycle and can make both conception and carrying a pregnancy to term a challenge. Estrogen dominance is not the only contributor to infertility and miscarriages, but it is a major factor.

#7 Water Retention and Bloating

Progesterone blocks the action of another hormone called aldosterone, which causes the body to store water in the presence of dehydration. Progesterone blocks aldosterone receptors and allows the body to release excess water.

This is why, when progesterone is low (estrogen dominance), there can be an influx of water and sodium into your cells, resulting in water retention, bloating and possibly high blood pressure.

Water retention is a common symptom of estrogen dominance. Most women have experienced a sudden weight gain leading up to their period. As a matter of fact, you may even have what you refer to as 'fat clothes' that you only wear during those two weeks before your period.

#8 Depression and Headaches/Migraines

At least 60% of migraines experienced by women are a result of estrogen dominance.

Estrogen causes swelling in the brain (which is the cause of most migraine headaches) the same way it does in the breasts (causing swollen and/or sore breasts). Estrogen can also deplete magnesium levels, which causes arteries to spasm.

Excess estrogen can also lead to a decrease in serotonin levels. Common physical symptoms of low serotonin are:

1. Gut and heart problems
2. Cravings for carbohydrates, alcohol and certain drugs
3. SAD (Seasonal Affective Disorder). You can usually tell if you have SAD because you will dislike the dark weather or have a distinct fall/winter depression.
4. Sleep Apnea
5. Menopausal and PMS mood-related problems
6. Obesity
7. Bulimia
8. Narcolepsy
9. Migraines, tension headaches or chronic daily headaches
10. Fibromyalgia
11. TMJ
12. Sleep challenges

#9 Decreased Sex Drive
Most women find their sex drive waxes and wanes with their cycle. However, when you are estrogen dominant, most women find the drive just isn't there at all.

#10 Heart Disease
Estrogen dominance promotes blood clotting and reduced vascular tone, which can lead to serious heart disease, including strokes and heart attacks.

If you are passing large blood clots during your period, then you are likely experiencing estrogen dominance. Being estrogen dominant is especially dangerous for women who have a history of heart disease in their family.

#11 Fatigue

Mitochondria are the cell's power producers: they convert energy into forms that are usable by the cell. Simply put, excess estrogen steals oxygen from mitochondria, and one result of less oxygen for your cells is fatigue.

Resources: www.raypeat.com

#12 Gallbladder Disease

Estrogen dominance thickens bile, which promotes gallbladder disease.

#13 Increased Risk of Autoimmune Disorders

Is it coincidental that autoimmune diseases such as Hashimoto's Thyroiditis, Lupus, Crohn's and Grave's disease are on the rise at the same time that estrogen dominance is also on the rise? This is definitely food for thought.

#14 Allergies

Elevated estrogen increases histamine release, causing red, itchy, inflamed tissues and gastrointestinal distress.

SUMMARY

Estrogen and progesterone are hormones that carry messages through your blood to target cells.

Estrogen is needed, but too much, relative to progesterone, is a problem known as estrogen dominance.

We know estrogen dominance can be directly or indirectly responsible for the following symptoms.

A printable list for you to check the following symptoms can be found at www.HormoneRollerCoaster.com

- Allergies
- Autoimmune disorders
- Bloating
- Blurred vision
- Constant worrying, unprovoked anxiety
- Constipation
- Cravings for carbohydrates or sweets
- Crying spells
- Decreased sex drive
- Depression
- Difficulty losing weight
- Drowsiness
- Endometriosis
- Faintness, dizziness, tremors and cold sweats
- Fatigue
- Feelings of fear or anxiety
- Fibrocystic breasts
- Forgetfulness, confusion
- Gallbladder disease
- Hair loss
- Headaches
- Heart attack risk
- Heart palpitations or rapid pulse
- Heavier, more frequent and more painful periods
- Heavy periods with or without blood clots
- Increased risk of breast cancer
- Increased risk of endometrial cancer
- Indecisiveness

- Infertility issues
- Insomnia
- Internal trembling
- Irritability
- Itching and crawling skin sensations
- Lack of concentration
- Lack of coordination
- Migraines
- Moodiness
- Muscle cramps and joint pain
- Muscle twitching and jerking
- Nervousness
- Nightmares
- Numbness
- Outbursts of temper
- Short menstrual cycles
- Sighing and yawning
- Sleepiness
- Sore, tender and/or swollen breasts
- Stroke risk
- Unjustified weight gain particularly around your abdomen, hips and thighs
- Uterine fibroids
- Water retention

Now that you know the symptoms associated with estrogen dominance, the next step is to lower your estrogen and raise your progesterone.

To do this, you need to correct the cause of your estrogen dominance. Since each woman is different, I am going to walk you step by step through the possibilities and help you identify which causes relate to you specifically, then outline the action steps you will to take.

CHAPTER 5

The First Step:
The Fast Track Foundation Overview

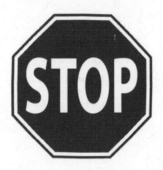

BEFORE PROCEEDING,
PLEASE MAKE SURE YOU HAVE READ

Chapter 1: Getting Started

Chapter 2: How the Book is Organized

Chapter 3: Do We Really Need Vitamins?

Chapter 4: Hormones 101

Because women lead such busy lives, I am giving you the **Fast Track Foundation** overview first so you can take immediate action. The overview will be followed by a more detailed explanation of each step.

Given that nutritional supplements are constantly changing, I have chosen not to list my recommended brands within the context of this book. My current supplement suggestions for the **Fast Track Founda-**

tion, along with all other nutritional supplement recommendations, can be found at www.HormoneRollerCoaster.com

#1. Supplement with Daily Essential Nutrients:
EVERYONE TAKES THIS STEP

You can't make a single hormone if you are deficient in even one mineral or one vitamin. Therefore, I have drawn on my 30-plus years of experience to design a list of essential nutrients that are required for daily supplementation to ensure that you aren't lacking in any key nutrient.

I will refer to this list of nutrients throughout the entire book as your Daily Essential Nutrients because I consider them to be an essential part of your daily life if you wish to achieve and maintain hormone balance.

The Daily Essential Nutrients make a strong foundation for your daily nutrient requirements, but I will be making suggestions for the temporary addition of specific targeted nutrients to address any area that is out of balance.

Once balance has been restored, most additional targeted nutrients can be stopped. However, I highly recommend that you always take your Daily Essential Nutrients.

#2. Supplement with Magnesium Citrate
MOST WOMEN WILL NEED TO TAKE THIS STEP

In my experience, women of all ages benefit immensely from taking magnesium over and above what is suggested in the Daily Essential Nutrients.

Magnesium is required for more than 300 reactions in your body. I could write dozens of chapters alone on the importance of magnesium for optimal health. However, we are Fast Tracking so all you need to know right now is the significance of magnesium deficiency for hormonal balance.

(a) You can't make ANY hormones without an adequate supply of magnesium.

All hormones are created from cholesterol and cholesterol cannot be made into hormones without magnesium.

(b) Magnesium acts like a spark plug for the adrenal glands and for the energy system of every cell in the body. Together with vitamin C and vitamin B5 (pantothenic acid), magnesium helps rejuvenate exhausted adrenal glands (details on adrenal glands are in chapter 10).

(c) Magnesium works with vitamin B6 to reduce estrogen and increase progesterone, which of course helps you reduce your estrogen dominance.

(d) Calcium causes muscles to contract and magnesium causes them to release. So any contracted states in your body, such as menstrual cramps, muscle tension or headaches/migraines, will respond favorably to magnesium.

(e) Another contracted state correlating with low levels of magnesium is improper elimination. Your body will try to eliminate excess estrogen through your bowels, but if your bowel does not empty properly, you will reabsorb the estrogen. This is another factor contributing to estrogen dominance (more details on proper bowel function in chapter 11).

#3 Supplement with B6 <u>and</u>/<u>or</u> Indole-3-Carbinol (I-3-C)
ALL WOMEN WILL NEED TO TAKE THIS STEP

(A) For Mild to Moderate Symptoms Choose Vitamin B6

Estrogen dominance usually results in a vitamin B6 (pyridoxine) deficiency. Taking supplemental B6 from ovulation to the first day of your period will help your liver clear excess estrogen from your body. B6 is also a necessary building block for progesterone.

The suggested amount is 200 mg of B6 (over and above what is in your Daily Essential Nutrients). It is critical that you take the B6 with your Daily Essential Nutrients. If you take any isolated B vitamin (such as B6) without taking the whole B complex family (as found in the Daily Essential Nutrients), you can cause an imbalance of B vitamins in your body.

Determining Approximate Times of Ovulation

Most women ovulate approximately 14 days before the first day of their period; so in order to work out when you ovulate, you'll need to do a bit of homework. It will be necessary to count the number of the days from the start of your period till the start of your next period. Let's say it is 25 days. Subtract 14 from this number and you'll get 11, which means that 11 days after the first day of your period you are likely to ovulate. Another example: From the start of one period to the start of the next is 30 days. Subtract 14 days from 30 and you get 16 days, which means that sixteen days from the start of your period you are probably ovulating.

Start taking your extra vitamin B6 from the day you ovulate and stop taking it when you start your period. Using it during this time frame will give you the best results. You don't need to stress about it though. If you are off by a day or two, it will not cause you any harm.

(B) For Severe Symptoms or Excessive Bleeding, Choose I-3-C

Your liver regulates your hormone balance by dumping excess hormones into your bowel to be excreted. Sometimes, for varying reasons, your liver does not do this very effectively. vitamin B6 can help, but when the symptoms are severe you will want to ensure the liver is metabolizing this excess estrogen efficiently. This is when I recommend Indole-3-Carbinol, called I-3-C for short.

If you have the following symptoms, I-3-C is a better choice for you than vitamin B6.

- severe hot flashes/night sweats
- endometriosis
- fibroids
- infertility
- prone to miscarriages
- hormonally induced migraines
- excessive heavy periods
- extreme menstrual cramping

I-3-C is a phytochemical isolated from cruciferous vegetables such as broccoli, cauliflower, Brussels sprouts, turnips, kale, green cabbage, mustard seed, etc. It reduces estrogen dominance symptoms by activating enzymes in the liver, which change excessive estrogen into harmless compounds for elimination.

The suggested amount is 200 mg twice a day. I-3-C is taken daily, as opposed to B6 which is only taken from ovulation to period.

Please note that pregnant women should not take I-3-C due to its modulation of estrogen. Also note it has a strong characteristic odor, which is lessened when stored in the refrigerator. It can be taken with or without food.

(C) You Can Choose Both

I generally suggest taking only one product or the other because I have found that most women prefer to take fewer, rather than more, supplements. However, if you have had long-term premenstrual issues or your symptoms are escalating, then there is no harm in taking both vitamin B6 (from ovulation to period) and I-3-C every day. In fact, it should speed up your results.

WHAT YOUR BASIC FAST TRACK FOUNDATION CHOICE A WILL LOOK LIKE

After Breakfast:
  Daily Essential Nutrients
  B6 200 mg (from ovulation to period)

Before Bed:
  450 mg of elemental magnesium from magnesium citrate

WHAT YOUR BASIC FAST TRACK FOUNDATION CHOICE B WILL LOOK LIKE

After Breakfast:
  Daily Essential Nutrients
  I-3-C 200 mg

After Lunch or Dinner:
  I-3-C 200 mg

Before Bed:
  450 mg of elemental magnesium from magnesium citrate

WHAT YOUR BASIC FAST TRACK FOUNDATION CHOICE C WILL LOOK LIKE

After Breakfast:
  Daily Essential Nutrients
  B6 200 mg (from ovulation to period)
  I-3-C 200 mg

After Lunch or Dinner:
  I-3-C 200 mg

Before Bed:
  450 mg of elemental magnesium from magnesium citrate

What Clients Have Said About The Fast Track Foundation

*I started taking the **Fast Track Foundation** at the WOW event. Within 4 days I no longer had hot flashes. They weren't severe or frequent but had returned after not having them for 3 years.*

I am no longer wearing my bite guard and my lower teeth that used to ache in the morning from grinding all night don't ache. My libido is on its way back from a hiatus to who knows where. Also within a week I noticed my nails were growing. I've been a nail biter all my life and I have nails! My skin is softer, less "chicken skin" on the backs of my upper arms and thighs. Thanks Brenda for your amazing gift of teaching nutrition and wellness.

–Monique M, Vancouver, BC

*I started on Brenda's recommended **Fast Track Foundation** and I quickly noticed improvements such as better sleep, calmer days, & a lessening of hot flashes.*

–Lumen, Nelson, BC

"The first wealth is health."

~Ralph Waldo Emerson

CHAPTER 6

Fast Track Solution One:
Daily Essential Nutrients

To get a printable copy of the Daily Essential Nutrients listed below visit www.HormoneRollerCoaster.com

You can certainly take more than the amounts listed below, but the following are the daily minimums I suggest.

- Vitamin A (Palmitate) 5,000 IU
- B1 (also called Thiamine) 30 mg
- B2 (also called Riboflavin) 30 mg
- B3 (also called niacin and niacinamide) 30 mg
- B5 (also called pantothenic acid) 35 mg
- B6 (also called pyridoxine) 30 mg
  Note: The best form of B6 is pyridoxal-5-phosphate (P-5-P) because it is ready to use. It does not need to be converted in your liver to the active form. Rarely do companies put P-5-P into their B complexes because it is the most expensive form. Therefore, look for a B complex with a combination of pyridoxine and P-5-P.
- Choline 25 mg
- Inositol 25 mg
- Paba (Paraminobenzoic acid) 15 mg
- Biotin 35 mcg
- Folic Acid 500 mcg

- Vitamin B12 35 mcg

- Calcium Ascorbate and bioflavanoids (total combined) 1,000 mg
  Note: Calcium Ascorbate is a buffered form of vitamin C. It is better tolerated, better absorbed and stays in your system longer. Ascorbic acid and time-release vitamin C are not recommended. Bioflavonoids are part of the C complex; in nature they are found in foods such as the white of an orange peel. Bioflavanoids allow the body to reap more benefits from vitamin C.

- Vitamin D3 500 IU

- Vitamin E (d-alpha tocopherol) 400 IU

- Calcium citrate 65 mg

- Magnesium citrate 65 mg

- Potassium citrate 25 mg

- Manganese citrate 1 mg

- Zinc citrate 5 mg

- Iodine (Kelp) 25 mcg

- Chromium HVP chelate 35 mcg

- Selenium HVP chelate 50 mcg

- Molybdenum citrate 25 mcg

- Boron Citrate 25 mcg

- Alfalfa Leaf Powder 350 mg
  (I suggest Alfalfa as it is the richest land source of trace minerals. However, you can substitute it and/or add more trace minerals by supplementing with algae, ionic minerals, bee pollen, and/or aloe vera juice.)

- Omega 3 EPA 180 mg DHA 120 mg

- Green Tea Extract (cathechin polyphenols) 400 mg

- MSM (methyl-sulfonyl-methane) 1,000 mg

To get all of the essential daily nutrients listed, you will likely need a bottle of each of the following.

1. A high quality multivitamin/mineral that includes alfalfa for the trace minerals (not listed). It will also have vitamin A, all the B's, vitamin D, all the minerals (listed)

2. Buffered vitamin C (called calcium ascorbate) with bioflavanoids.

3. Vitamin E

4. MSM

5. Omega 3

6. Green Tea Extract

KEY BENEFITS OF THE ESSENTIAL DAILY NUTRIENTS

Vitamin A is needed for lustrous hair, healthy nails and beautiful skin, plus great eyesight.

B Complex is needed by the nervous system. Without it, you can become senile, depressed, suffer with memory loss and have issues with focus and concentration.

B complex increases your energy and metabolism, calms your nerves, and improves your sleep and complexion.

It is critical for the function of your adrenal glands (you will discover the significance of your adrenal glands in chapter 10).

Vitamin C plays an integral role in making all of your hormones including estrogen, progesterone and testosterone.

It helps form strong bones and collagen, which keeps your cells together. If you maintain high levels of vitamin C, you can prevent, minimize and even reverse wrinkling.

Vitamin C helps keep your adrenal glands strong, and helps your body break down and absorb iron.

Research shows that vitamin C is effective in preventing cancers of the breast, cervix, colon, rectum, esophagus, larynx, lung, mouth, prostate and stomach, alleviating its symptoms, and, in some cases, halting its progress.

Vitamin D helps place calcium in the bones and protects against depression.

Vitamin E is most known to help menstruating and peri-menopausal women with breast tenderness, mood swings, anxiety, confusion, and headaches.

Macro and Trace Minerals

Calcium, potassium, zinc and magnesium are known as macro-minerals because they are present in relatively high amounts in body tissues. They are measured in milligrams (mg). Other minerals such as chromium, iodine, selenium, and vanadium are termed micro or trace minerals and are measured in micrograms (mcg).

These trace minerals are so small that no one seems to pay much attention to them, but your body relies on both macro and trace minerals to generate billions of tiny electrical impulses. Without these impulses, not a single muscle, including your heart, would be able to function.

Here are just a few examples of what minerals do.

Both **macro** and **trace minerals** are essential for rejuvenating your adrenal glands.

Zinc, **Iodine** and **Selenium** are needed for healthy thyroid function.

Chromium helps balance your blood sugar.

Omega-3 works to turn on the genes that burn body fat and turn off the genes that store it. Omega-3 supports thyroid function, improves your moods, increases mental alertness, and reduces your fat cravings.

Green Tea Extract is for mega-antioxidant protection. Plus it helps increase brain power and your metabolism for higher energy and fat-burning abilities.

MSM (methyl-sulfonyl-methane) is one of my absolute favorite nutrients, as it helps regenerate all body tissues. It has the ability to reduce pain and inflammation, allergic reactions and headaches. It also facilitates blood sugar balancing. MSM allows all cells to be more permeable, flexible and elastic (allowing nutrients into cells, including your hormones, and flushing toxins out). When combined with vitamin C, it does amazing work to keep your skin young, and wrinkle free!

Supplement Selection

At www.HormoneRollerCoaster.com you will find my current brand recommendations for supplements, as well as my complimentary comprehensive consumer report called "Don't Flush Your Money Down the Toilet! Learn the Difference Between Quality and Hype!"

This report will be an invaluable tool for putting your vitamin regime together. Choosing the right supplements is way more complicated than you might think. It would take years of research for you to learn the details I have provided for you in my report. I urge you to print a copy of my report and study it. Then take it with you when you go supplement shopping so you don't make the common errors most people make.

I would rather you buy nothing than flush your money down the toilet on poor quality supplements.

"The doctor of the future
will no longer treat the
human frame with
drugs, but rather will cure
and prevent disease
with nutrition."

~Thomas Edison

CHAPTER 7

Fast Track Solution Two:
Magnesium, The Miracle Mineral

The **Fast Track Foundation Overview** explained why you must have an ample supply of magnesium if you want to have optimal hormone balance.

Each person is unique in their requirements, so this chapter will help you decide whether you need to be taking extra magnesium, how much you should be taking and when you no longer require additional supplementation.

You do need to understand this section because you can't rely on blood tests to inform you.

The body of an adult human contains approximately 25 to 30 grams of magnesium. Of this, the greatest part is deposited in the bones; much is also found in the muscles, liver, brain, kidneys and in the blood.

Given the amount of magnesium in your blood is only $1/10$ of what is in your cells, testing your blood to see if your cells have enough magnesium is useless.

Fortunately for you, your symptoms are the best indicator of whether or not you need to supplement with magnesium.

If your body requires magnesium, you will likely have at least a couple of the following common symptoms.

- Loose/sensitive teeth
- Depression
- Poor co-ordination
- Anxiety
- Easy startle response
- Irritable nerves or muscles
- Nervous tics or twitches
- Spasms, tremors, convulsions, or seizures
- Irregular heartbeat, tachycardia
- Painful and cold hands or feet
- Excessive body odor
- Dimmed vision
- Apprehensiveness, confusion, disorientation
- Nausea, dizziness, or light-headedness
- Feel constantly cold
- Hypersensitivity to noise
- Personality changes
- Loss of appetite
- Muscle pain and/or fibromyalgia

Of course, any of these could be symptoms of other issues. However, if you have just one of the symptoms in the questionnaire following, it is almost certain that you need to supplement with magnesium.

____ Very definite and strong craving for chocolate

____ History of kidney stones

____ High blood pressure (or take high blood pressure medications)

____ Clench your jaw or grind your teeth or wear a night guard to protect your teeth

____ Menstrual cramps

____ Tension headaches or migraines

____ Muscle cramps

____ Angina

____ Asthma

____ A lot of muscle tension

To get a printable copy of these symptoms and the questionnaire, visit www.HormoneRollerCoaster.com

Here are three examples of what your questionnaire could look like if you needed to supplement with magnesium.

Sample A

____ Do you have a very definite and strong craving for chocolate

____ Do you have a history of kidney stones

____ Do you have high blood pressure (or take high blood pressure medications)

_X_ Do you clench your jaw or grind your teeth or wear a night guard to protect your teeth

_X_ Do you get menstrual cramps

____ Do you get tension headaches or migraines

____ Do you get muscle cramps

____ Do you have angina

____ Do you have asthma

_X_ Do you get a lot of muscle tension

Sample B

____ Do you have a very definite and strong craving for chocolate

_X_ Do you have a history of kidney stones

___ Do you have high blood pressure (or take high blood pressure medications)

___ Do you clench your jaw or grind your teeth or wear a night guard to protect your teeth.

___ Do you get menstrual cramps

_X_ Do you get tension headaches or migraines

_X_ Do you get muscle cramps

___ Do you have angina

___ Do you have asthma

___ Do you get a lot of muscle tension

Sample C

_X_ Do you have a very definite and strong craving for chocolate

___ Do you have a history of kidney stones

___ Do you have high blood pressure (or take high blood pressure medications)

___ Do you clench your jaw or grind your teeth or wear a night guard to protect your teeth.

___ Do you get menstrual cramps

___ Do you get tension headaches or migraines

___ Do you get muscle cramps

___ Do you have angina

_X_ Do you have asthma

___ Do you get a lot of muscle tension

Suggested Dosages

A good start would be at least 400 mg elemental magnesium, or three capsules of my recommended brand, taken any time after eight p.m. (before bed is generally an easy time to remember, especially if you leave your bottle of magnesium next to your bed).

If after two weeks your magnesium symptoms are not lessening, try approximately 540 mg of elemental magnesium before bed.

If after another two weeks your magnesium deficiency symptoms still aren't lessening, then try approximately 670 mg of elemental magnesium before bed.

If any dosage causes your stool to become extremely loose, then cut back by one capsule.

** IMPORTANT NOTE. *In the event you don't have time to read my entire report "Don't Flush Your Money Down the Toilet, Learn the Difference Between Quality and Hype!" or you don't use my recommended brands, it is important to know that most supplement manufacturers will only list the weight of the magnesium and not the elemental amount. So, if in the ingredient listing, it doesn't say "magnesium from magnesium citrate" then you are likely looking at the weight of the capsule and not the actual amount of absorbable magnesium you are getting.*

Other Forms of Magnesium

While other forms of magnesium are available, I prefer magnesium citrate. I researched quite extensively before recommending magnesium citrate to my clients. There are lots of studies on the absorption of magnesium, including one from the University of Maryland Medical Center that reports, "magnesium citrate is a compound of magnesium carbonate and citric acid and it is one of the more readily absorbable supplementary forms of this key mineral."

When the "newest kid on the block," magnesium bisglycinate, arrived, I did a trial with my client base. Although the benefits looked great on paper, this product just did not deliver the consistent results I was looking for, plus it was more expensive. Now you can't convince me to use anything but magnesium citrate.

Put Your Calcium Aside

Given that the focus is on increasing magnesium levels, I suggest you put away any calcium supplements you are currently taking.

1. You are getting an absorbable form of calcium in your Daily Essentials.
2. By taking additional magnesium, you will be better utilizing the calcium you get from your diet.

Please do not try to compensate with extra dairy products. You do not need to load up on calcium to make your bones strong. In fact, I guarantee that the more calcium you ingest, the more health issues you will have. For your free report called "Important Facts That Can Make or 'Break' Your Bones" visit www.HormoneRollerCoaster.com

Do You Need Supplemental Magnesium Forever?

Once all your symptoms have disappeared, try cutting your dosage back by 1 capsule. Maintain that new dosage for at least two weeks. If your symptom(s) reappear, then increase your dosage again. If you still do not have any magnesium symptoms after two weeks at the reduced dosage, then cut back again by 1 capsule. If the reduced dosage causes your symptom(s) to reappear, go back to your previous dosage.

You will keep maintaining the next lower dosage for a minimum of two weeks before cutting back again, always increasing to your previous dosage if symptoms reappear. You will continue this process until you are no longer taking the magnesium.

Some women will never have to take supplemental magnesium again, while other women find that every time they reduce or stop their dosage, symptoms return, so they feel best when they remain on magnesium supplements. There will also be women who find they need to take magnesium periodically throughout their life.

If at any time you get a recurrence of symptoms, simply return to taking supplemental magnesium.

How Do You Become Deficient in Magnesium?

- The more calcium you take in through supplements and diet, the more you diminish your magnesium absorption
- Low dietary intakes: the best sources of magnesium are leafy green vegetables such as spinach, kale and Swiss chard, which are sadly lacking from the typical diet
- The use of diuretics causes you to excrete magnesium
- Excess sweating depletes magnesium and other mineral levels in the body
- Drinking too much water flushes out magnesium and other minerals
- The more stress you are under, the more magnesium you will dump from your body
- Menstruating women tend to lose even more magnesium in the time-frame between ovulation and their period

That Chocolate Craving

Have you ever noticed that your craving for chocolate intensifies pre-period? Note that this type of craving is different than a craving for sugar and candy bars made with heavily sweetened milk chocolate. Dark chocolate (at least 70%) is a source of magnesium, which is why, if you are lacking in magnesium, you crave it. Remember though, this is not the recommended way to get your magnesium.

If you really need to indulge in chocolate, then skip the candy aisle and spend the money on a bar of good quality organic dark chocolate. The darker the better, as it will have more magnesium, plus antioxidants and "feel good" nutrients. The darker it is, the less sugar it contains, which is a bonus. Be careful though, as it will have more caffeine as well. The best part is you only need a small square or two to feel satisfied (at least that is all I am recommending you consume).

Here is What Some of My Clients Have to Say About Magnesium

Hi Brenda - I want to let you know a couple of things I'm very happy about. I started taking three magnesium before bed about 4 or 5 nights ago, & I have waited a few days to let you know this but two things have happened, almost immediately, which I thought was maybe just a fluke, but now that it is consistent for 5 days I'm sure it is the result of the magnesium. One, my stiffness is virtually gone! Whereas I used to be very creaky & stiff first thing in the morning, or if I sat for as little as 20 minutes driving to work, it is just - gone! The other amazing thing that is - gone! - is my chocolate craving. I had been into it again in a pretty bad way (thus my weight gain) & this week I just am not interested. This is the most amazing thing!

–Bonnie G, Red Deer, Alta

About two months ago at your suggestion my 19 year old daughter started taking 3 Magnesium capsules before bed to help soften her stool. It is working really well, no more painful b.m.s thank you!

–Susan M, Vancouver, BC

Hi Brenda- I attended your last all day seminar - the magnesium has changed my life!!! It is my new best friend!! I am telling all my friends about it. I am on disability for 20 migraines/month - cannot work on maternity - which is what I was put on earth to do. Since taking the magnesium - I take 6 a day - I no longer have tight shoulder muscles in spasms. I have the same number of migraines but much reduced in intensity. I have tried everything known to man for this migraine problem of 25 plus years - had even tried magnesium before, but maybe not the right kind or not enough. Perhaps I will be able to go back to work in time. Yours in gratitude.

–Kathie D, Drumheller, Alta

So I did what you suggested Sunday and have been taking 3 magnesium capsules at night before bed, and WOW! I cannot believe what incredible sleeps I have been having! I never would have thought that I had any sleep problems, but considering how incredibly good and well rested - like never before - that I have been feeling these past two mornings, I must have.

–Jody B, Calgary, Alta

"No disease that
can be treated by diet
should be treated
with any other means."

~Maimonides

CHAPTER 8

Fast Track Solution Three:
Vitamin B6 and I-3-C

You have all the information you need on these two nutrients in the **Fast Track Foundation Overview**, other than how to use them long-term.

You can safely take vitamin B6 until you stop having periods altogether. Even then you could continue, but there would be no point. The key is to always take it with the complete B complex family (as found in the Daily Essential Nutrients) or you will cause an imbalance of B vitamins in your body.

If your periods are all over the map, making it difficult for you to know when you ovulate, you can take B6 every day and just stop taking it while you have your period. If a pattern emerges, then begin using it from ovulation to period.

Some women will have more success with P-5-P (pyridoxal-5-phosphate) which is the active form of B6. If you choose P-5-P you would take 100 mg from the approximate date of ovulation (about 14 days preceding your period) to the day you start your period.

I-3-C (Indole-3-Carbinol)

I ask my clients this: "If I-3-C were free and/or tasted like chocolate, would you take it for the rest of your life?" The answer is always yes. I wish I could make it so because I know from experience that estrogen dominance is the greatest risk factor for breast cancer and the best supplemental protection against estrogen dominance is I-3-C.

If you want to get down to a bare-bones supplement regime, then I would suggest you stay on the I-3-C for three months past the first cycle that feels balanced to you. Then cut down to 1 capsule of I-3-C per day for three months. Then, if you still feel your hormones are in balance, you can stop taking the I-3-C altogether.

If you have a history of breast cancer in your family, or if you have any lumps or adhesions that are concerning you, I would highly recommend making I-3-C a permanent part of your Daily Essential Nutrients supplement regime.

CHAPTER 9

Fast Track Solution Four:
Eliminate Candida Overgrowth

What happens when you are suffering from a collection of seemingly unrelated symptoms and yet all the blood tests you've had indicate that there is nothing wrong with you?

Is it all in your head? Definitely not! You could have an undetected problem known as a Candida overgrowth or Candidiasis.

What The Heck is a Candida Overgrowth?

You might have heard of Candida in the context of a vaginal yeast infection, but the Candida I am talking about is the one that changes from a yeast to a fungus within your intestinal tract and spreads like wildfire.

Everyone has this yeast we call Candida, living in harmony with other microbes within the intestines. We have "good bacteria" that keep this Candida yeast in check. In small populations, Candida yeast isn't harmful, but when allowed to proliferate into a condition called Candidiasis, the symptoms can become anywhere from mildly annoying to severely debilitating.

For the sake of simplicity, I am going to refer to a Candida overgrowth or Candidiasis, as simply 'Candida' throughout the remainder of this book.

How Do You Get Candida?

Antibiotics were a great discovery and have been used to effectively kill off different varieties of unwanted or dangerous bacteria; but when used indiscriminately (for non-threatening illnesses), they also kill off your protective "good bacteria," which allows the Candida to take hold of your intestines.

Antibiotics, both oral and through your food supply, aren't the only enemy of friendly bacteria.

Other Contributing Factors

- When your hormone system is disrupted ie: birth control pills alter the body's hormonal balance and pregnancies temporarily change normal hormone cycles
- High-sugar diets feed the yeast, causing it to multiply even faster
- An alkaline/acid imbalance provides just the right environment to encourage the growth of yeast
- Cortisone and prednisone suppress the immune system, allowing the opportunistic yeast to take over
- Radiation and chemotherapy kill friendly bacteria
- Most surgery calls for antibiotics, plus surgery is a huge stress. Either factor leaves you susceptible to Candida

That Darn Stress!

When you become stressed, your body releases more of a hormone called cortisol. This hormone can weaken the immune system, and at the same time, cause elevated levels of blood sugar. Since yeast feeds off of sugar, it is able to grow much quicker than normal in this environment.

What Are The Symptoms of Candida?

Symptoms vary from person to person. While one person may only have one or two, another may have them all. Some of the typical symptoms of Candida include: foggy brain, allergies, skin problems, hormonal imbalances, poor memory, poor concentration, fatigue, intestinal gas, bloating, abdominal fullness, heartburn, acid reflux, gastritis, trouble sleeping, and constipation or diarrhea, or both alternating.

In order of importance, Candida is the next fast track solution to address because:

1. It can be the root cause of almost any health symptom from joint pain to indigestion.
2. Candida gobbles up your progesterone, leading to severe estrogen dominance.
3. If you have Candida, you can swallow all the supplements you want, exercise like a demon, eat all organic food and meditate on a mountain top, but you won't balance your hormones until you eliminate that excess Candida.

Therefore, it is imperative you figure out whether or not you have Candida; and if you do, you must use my six-pronged approach to treat it before you can effectively move forward in balancing your hormones.

Who Can Diagnose You?

You can. In fact, you must diagnose yourself because some doctors still refuse to admit that Candida can overgrow in the intestines and cause illness. This is due partly to the lack of agreement over a definitive diagnostic test for intestinal yeast overgrowth. And it is partly due to the fact that your doctor is trained in surgery and medication, but he/she is not likely trained in nutritional approaches to health.

Until a definitive diagnostic test is developed, it is wise to look at evidence from different sources to give you a good idea of whether you have a yeast overgrowth or not.

What I recommend is the symptomatology method which includes:

1. Looking at your medical history
2. Evaluating your own symptoms and energy
3. Doing the home spit test

I have found the symptomatology method to be exceptionally accurate. There are tests for Candida offered by holistic practitioners (which are not 100% accurate) that cost over one hundred dollars to conclude the same thing you can conclude for free. If you use the symptomatology method, you can use the money you saved to purchase the supplements you require to treat the Candida overgrowth.

The Four Step Symptomatology Method

This method involves answering three sets of questions and performing something called a "spit test." Once you have completed all four steps, you can determine whether or not Candida is an underlying issue for you or not.

To print a copy of the three sets of questions used in the Four Step Symptomatology Method please visit www.HormoneRollerCoaster.com

Step One: Have An Honest Look At Your Medical History

How many times (to the best of your recollection) have you had antibiotics?

0-5 times ___ 5-10 times ___ 10-20 times ___ Over 20 times ___

Have you ever been on birth control pills?

Have you ever been pregnant?

Have you ever eaten a high-sugar diet?

Have you ever tested your pH balance and found it was acidic?

Have you ever had cortisone or prednisone?

Have you ever had radiation?

Have you ever had surgery?

Have you ever experienced an intense period of high stress?

Ask yourself the above questions only to establish whether or not Candida could potentially be a problem for you. The more "yes" answers you give, the more likely you are to have developed Candida. You must complete the next three steps and then look at the entire evidence, not just pieces of it, to draw your final conclusion.

Step Two: Evaluate Your Symptoms

Candida affects each person differently. No two people have identical symptoms, but the following questionnaire highlights the symptoms most commonly associated with Candida.

An important note: You can have <u>vaginal yeast infections</u> and not have Candida and you can have Candida and not get vaginal yeast infections. However, if you have repeated vaginal yeast infections, then you should be suspicious of Candida.

Complete the following quiz by putting an x in the blank for any symptoms that currently apply to you.

1. Do you form gas or bloat when you eat? ____

2. Do you have acid reflux, heartburn or gastritis? ____

3. Are you prone to constipation or diarrhea or both? ____

4. Do you have an itchy nose? ____

5. Do you have ear sensitivity/ringing/itching or fluid in your ears? ____

6. Do you have a dry mouth? ____

7. Are you hypothyroid or suffer with cold hands or feet? ____

8. Do you have brain fog, which causes you to have trouble thinking clearly, poor memory or poor concentration? ____

9. Do you suffer from fatigue for no reason? ____

10. Does your vision get blurry, then clear, then blurry? ___

11. Are you hypoglycemic? Indicated by being shaky or irritable if late for a meal, sleepy after a meal, or sweaty during sleep? ___

12. Do you have deep pains in your legs, arms and back? ___

13. Do you have cravings for sugar, carbohydrates or alcohol? ___

14. Do you suffer with continuous or repeated vaginal burning, itching, or discharge? ___

15. Do you have depression, anxiety, or loss of interest and/or pleasure? ___

16. Do you have trouble sleeping? ___

17. Do you have numbness, burning or tingling in any of your body parts? ___

Total Score: _____

If you have a total of 4 or more symptoms, consider Candida a possibility.

Step Three: Rate Your Energy Level

On a scale of 0 to 10, zero is *shoot me I might as well be dead*, and 10 is an achievable level of energy.

Current energy _____

Fatigue, rated at 7 or less, is the only symptom common to each person with Candida. If you score 8, 9 or 10, it is unlikely that your symptoms are related to Candida. If you score an 8, 9, or 10 for part of the day and 7 and below for the rest of the day, then you likely have a low blood sugar problem.

If your energy goes up and down within a day, but doesn't go any higher than a 7, you could have both low blood sugar (hypoglycemia) and Candida.

People with Candida really struggle with their energy and the ability to feel well. Those with low blood sugar may have swings of energy levels but generally only have varying periods of feeling unwell.

Step Four: Do the Candida Home Spit Test

First thing in the morning, before you put ANYTHING in your mouth, get a clear glass. Fill with filtered water and work up a bit of saliva, then spit it into the glass of water. Check the water every 15 minutes or so for up to one hour without touching the glass. If you have Candida, you will see strings (like legs) traveling down into the water from the saliva floating on the top, or "cloudy" saliva will sink to the bottom of the glass, or cloudy specks will seem to be suspended in the water. If there are no strings and the saliva is still floating after at least one hour, then you don't likely have Candida.

The spit test is not foolproof and should not be used as your primary decision-making tool but it is an excellent guideline when paired with the other symptoms you may have.

Additional Information for Consideration

It is common for people with Candida to:

1. Be sensitive to tobacco smoke, perfumes, insecticides, fabric shop odors and other chemicals.

2. Feel worse on damp, muggy days or in moldy places.

3. Have moderate, severe or persistent athlete's foot, ringworm, jock itch or other chronic fungous infections of the skin or nails.

4. Crave sugar, bread or alcoholic beverages.

5. Get minimal results from taking nutritional supplements.

6. Have multiple health concerns that seem totally unrelated.

7. Struggle to feel well.

8. Not find a medical reason for their health concerns.

DECISION TIME

You must evaluate all four of these steps together. You cannot make a decision based on just one of the four.

For example, as a child I had many rounds of antibiotics, and from the ages of 16 to 25 I had been on birth control pills. For a good part of those years I also ate a high-sugar diet. Therefore, my perimenopausal symptoms could have been related to Candida.

As I carried on through the steps, I discovered I didn't have any of the typical symptoms and my energy always correlated to the amount of sleep I had. Someone with Candida will only benefit a little or not at all from a good night's sleep. I also passed my spit test. If I had based my decision solely on my answers in step one, I would have thought I had Candida. But my conclusion after completing all four steps was that I did not have Candida.

If you believe your medical history has set you up for the possibility of Candida, and you have four or more symptoms, with 7 or less energy and a failed spit test, then it is extremely likely you have Candida.

Still Not Sure?

My six-pronged approach to eliminating Candida is such a healthy program, you will benefit from it whether you have Candida or not. In other words, it won't hurt and can only help you.

If you choose not to do the Candida Program when you truly have Candida, you will notice that no matter what you do in terms of exercise, diet or supplements, you will struggle to feel great and you really won't see much improvement in your hormonal symptoms.

When you have Candida, the only thing that will make an extensive difference in how you feel is eliminating the Candida. So if you decide not to do the Candida program, you can proceed to the next fast track solution and then re-evaluate your health symptoms in six to eight weeks. If your symptoms have not improved, then I would reconsider doing the Candida Program, regardless of your original diagnosis.

WHAT YOU SHOULD KNOW

Candida Yeast Is Tenacious.

It won't leave without a fight. Many people have tried very restricted diets in hopes of choking off the Candida's food supply and killing it. This might provide temporary relief, but soon after these people return to normal eating, their health starts to take a downturn again.

If you have treated Candida in the past, you might think you are protected. In my experience, most people have not learned how to treat Candida in a way that kills the overgrowth and prevents it from returning. If you start experiencing new or old health problems months after your Candida Program, it is very likely you have Candida again.

Do You Want Your Life Back?

The women who have been lucky enough to discover and successfully treat their Candida with my six-pronged approach now have their lives back and their hormones balanced!

Here Are Just a Few Testimonials

My 24 yr. old daughter is starting week 4 tomorrow of your Candida Program. She can't remember the last time she felt this great. She is no longer having problems with insomnia and PMS.... no longer feeling depressed..... no longer having headaches..... the pain that she has had for years in her hip is gone... and she can now sleep on her side again.... she has also started working out again...... my going to your workshop has changed her life... and I don't think that there are words that can justly express my gratitude to you.

–Marilyn A, Coquitlam, BC

Despite taking hundreds of dollars worth of supplements every month for over 12 years, I was constantly under the weather and battling hormonal issues. I learned from you that I was battling a major Candida infestation for at least 15 years – perhaps longer. It was the result of being on anti-biotics for an extended period of time trying to deal with a bacterial infection. Well, I have been on your Candida program for less than a month and I am now in the best health I have been in since December 1991.

–Lee P, Victoria, BC

I started your Candida program cleanse just over a week ago, and I cannot believe the difference. My energy is back to where it used to be, and I am remembering things I didn't even know I'd forgotten. I'm clearer and more able to deal with stress - of which there is a lot, like so many other people. thank you thank you!

–Shannon E, Pemberton, BC

TREATING CANDIDA

There are hundreds of programs available for treating Candida. Selections can be found at most health food stores or through any holistic health care provider.

For 100% success, make sure any program you embark on follows my entire six-pronged approach.

OVERVIEW OF MY SIX-PRONGED APPROACH
HOW TO ERADICATE CANDIDA IN 4 to 6 WEEKS

Step 1. Starve the Candida

The only food Candida can survive on is sugar, in all of its various forms. It does not feed on other yeast or fermented food. Many diets will have you exclude yeast and vinegars on the theory yeast promotes yeast. Although you may feel more bloated or tired when you consume yeast or vinegar, it does <u>not</u> cause the yeast to grow.

Knowing this, the most critical dietary factor is to abstain from all refined sugar and grains. You must also avoid all other sources of sugar such as honey, molasses, all syrups, juices, soda, alcohol, cookies, cakes, candies, etc. In the critical stages, even natural sugars from fruit and high carbohydrate foods, such as whole grains, must be restricted.

Do not assume you know what you can and cannot eat. My program is MUCH more lenient than other programs but also MUCH more effective. It is very easy to follow, but you MUST adhere to the diet. This is not a typical weight loss diet where you can "cheat" and get back on track the next day. If you "cheat" on this program's diet, you will set yourself back by days or even weeks.

If you decide to put your own program together, follow a low-glycemic and low-carbohydrate diet.

Step 2 (a). Eradicate the Excess Candida

I have tried many of the available products for eradicating excess Candida and have found blended products give the best effect.

The product I am currently recommending in my program is a combination of:

> Pau D'Arco
>
> Grapefruit Seed Extract Concentrate
>
> Caprylic Acid
>
> Odorless Garlic
>
> Black Walnut Hulls
>
> Oregano Extract Powder

I suggest clients start slowly with their dosage; for example, with this particular product, only 1 capsule twice a day and increase as tolerated to 2 to 3 capsules three times a day.

What do I mean by 'as tolerated'?

Candida is constantly releasing toxins into your system, but when they die, they release their toxins all at once, causing a temporary worsening of symptoms. This reaction is referred to as "die-off," also known as the "Herxheimer reaction."

Die off generally doesn't last too long. It can feel like the flu, either mild with a few symptoms such as headaches or body aches, or severe where you feel very ill and may need bed rest for a day or two. You might just feel a little under the weather or no worse than a typical bad day for you. Some people do not feel anything at all. The key is to kill the Candida as quickly as possible but be able to cope with your symptoms at the same time.

Step 2 (b). Extra Insurance: Silver Solution

Please Note**If you are allergic to silver jewelry, you should patch test the inside of your arm to make sure you will not have an allergic reaction to silver. It is rare but it can happen.

It can be a more difficult process and take longer than expected to eradicate Candida if the infestation is heavy and/or has thrived for many years. This is why I have added the silver solution to the program. It decreases the length of time needed for treating the Candida and is instrumental in eradicating difficult-to-treat Candida.

I suggest adding 2 teaspoons twice a day, once the full dosage of "Candida Eradicator" capsules has been reached. Just take it directly into your mouth. It does not need to be diluted in anything. It can go before food or after food. It doesn't matter.

There are many liquid silver products on the market and most people think of them as "colloidal silver" but the one I recommend is far superior, because it is actually a silver solution and has been scientifically proven to be three times more effective as any other silver product. It is also 100% safe.

1. This silver solution will not accumulate in your body like other colloidal or ionic silver preparations. You will not turn blue, even if you drink a bottle every day for years. It passes through the body unchanged, producing no dangerous metabolites and is 99% cleared by the next day.

2. This specific silver solution holds three patents, which means it has been scientifically proven time and time again.

3. Unlike traditional antibiotics, it does not cause bacteria to mutate or become resistant to it, producing super bugs such as MRSA (Methicillin-Resistant Staphylococcus Aureus).

4. This silver solution kills viruses, bacteria, yeasts (Candida), fungus and molds such as MRSA, Staph, avian influenza A, pneumonia, food poisoning, salmonella, E. coli, human papillomavirus (HPV), hepatitis, AIDS, SARS and malaria.

5. It does not destroy your friendly intestinal flora.

6. It does not interfere with the action of antibiotics or other drugs.

Step 3. Replenish Your Natural Healthy Intestinal Bacteria

Many women now know to take "good bacteria" or probiotics after a course of antibiotics. But, it makes me very sad when I hear they are wasting their money on inferior bacteria products. The majority of commercial bacteria (probiotic) products do not contain what the labels claim, or worse, contain no viable bacteria at all, or they do not have the proper bacteria required for your intestinal tract.

If you have relied on yogurt for your friendly bacteria, you likely will not have fared any better, because when fruit is added to yogurt, it destroys the bacteria. (Pasteurization of dairy products also limits the culture of live bacteria in yogurt, even if it is unsweetened.) There are many different kinds of bacteria, but only a few strains will provide the benefits you're looking for; yet yogurt labels rarely tell you exactly which strain of bacteria is in the product.

The three main kinds of beneficial bacteria are, in order of importance:

- Bifidobacteria
- Lactobacillus acidophilus
- Lactobacillus bulgaricus

Are You Getting the Right Bacteria?

Though acidophilus is the beneficial bacteria most people are familiar with, bifidobacteria are the most significant microorganisms in the small and large intestine. There are benefits to be had from acidophilus and bulgaricus, and they should be part of your beneficial bacteria supplement regime, but the bifidobacteria are the most important of these probiotics.

In order to successfully supplement and develop your healthy bacteria, you need a bacteria product with large amounts of bifidobacteria, as well as lactobacillus acidophilus and lactobacillus bulgaricus. The bacteria need to be resistant to heat to allow it to survive the journey through the stomach into the small intestine before being activated. The best bacteria will be sealed in individual packets because exposure to air will kill these good bacteria. Bacteria sealed in capsules will also lose potency due to the moisture from the capsules.

You must "implant" lots of friendly bacteria into your intestines or the Candida will have a greater chance of re-establishing itself.

Please make sure you get the right bacteria to do the job! Do not rely on advertising campaigns to persuade you. Make sure to get the type of bacteria product I have described. I suggest taking one full dosage in the morning, preferably before you eat, and again in the evening before bed.

Step 4. Supply All Nutrients for Healing

The great news is the Daily Essential Nutrients will give you all the nutrients you need both during and after your Candida Program.

Here are just a FEW of the nutrients found in the Daily Essential Nutrients and why they are perfect as a component of any Candida treatment:

- MSM (methyl-sulfonyl-methane) helps flush out the toxins created by the Candida (and more are created in the initial phase of the Candida cleanse known as the 'die-off' or 'Herxheimer reaction').

- Alfalfa is the richest land source of trace minerals. This helps keep your body from becoming too acidic.

- Vitamin A helps repair the mucous membranes of your intestinal tract.

- B vitamins support your nervous system.

- Omega 3 from salmon oil has strong antifungal properties.

- Buffered vitamin C with bioflavanoids protects against viral and bacterial infections.

- A balance of the vitamins/minerals strengthens the immune system.

Step 5. Boost Your Immune System

The primary function of the immune system is to protect the body against infection and the development of abnormal cells, or cancer. It is critical to repair a compromised immune system that has been damaged from toxins produced by a Candida overgrowth.

By taking a combination of the Daily Essential Nutrients and the right "Candida Eradicator" product, you will get the support you need to help restore your immune system. The added silver solution, while not directly boosting your immune system, will definitely be working to kill off any infections and viruses you may encounter, thus giving your immune system some needed relief.

Step 6. Ensure Healthy Elimination

Proper bowel function is critical for eliminating the toxins released during the Candida die-off and disposing of excess estrogen. When waste does not get eliminated efficiently, an ideal breeding ground for unwanted bacteria, yeast and parasites is created.

By following the **Fast Track Foundation**, you will already be well on your way to better bowel function. Many cases of improper elimination relate back to not enough magnesium. This problem has been remedied in the **Fast Track Foundation** because it includes supplemental magnesium.

HERE IS WHAT YOUR CANDIDA PROGRAM WILL LOOK LIKE

Before Breakfast:
 One dosage of friendly bacteria

After Breakfast:
 Daily Essential Nutrients
 B6 200 mg from ovulation to period **and/or**
 I-3-C 200 mg daily
 1-3 capsules of "Candida Eradicator"
 Add 2 teaspoons of silver solution when max dose of "Candida Eradicator" is reached

After Lunch:
 1-3 capsules of "Candida Eradicator"

After Dinner:
 I-3-C 200 mg (only if you are taking I-3-C as well as B6 or instead of B6)
 1-3 capsules of "Candida Eradicator"
 Add 2 teaspoons of silver solution when max dose of "Candida Eradicator" is reached

Before Bed:
 400 to 700 mg of elemental magnesium from magnesium citrate, plus one dosage of friendly bacteria

---

For details on my Candida Program, visit:
www.HormoneRollerCoaster.com

Is All of This Really Worth It?

My clients who have completed a Candida program think so. Here's what some of them have to say.

Being chronically 'sick' most of my life (not realizing it wasn't 'normal') my chronic fatigue/adrenal fatigue, hormone/perimenopausal issues, & a whole host of 'other' chronic issues were amplified by mercury poisoning 10 yrs ago.

*Two years ago, I started on Brenda's recommended **Fast Track Foundation**. I saw improvements such as better sleep, calmer days, & a lessening of hot flashes. HOWEVER, I was STILL plagued by extreme digestive & perimenopausal issues and had tried every Candida program out there, so was skeptical about trying yet 'another' one...*

OMG! Started Brenda's Candida program at the beginning of this year and I'm starting to feel like I did when I was in my 20's!!! More energy & vitality, I'm sleeping through the night (no hot flashes anymore), digestion / hormone balance is getting better, AND the best side-benefit is I've lost over 30 POUNDS!!!

If ANYONE has suffered with Candida, it's me. So if anyone else out there is suffering with this, PLEASE don't wait to do Brenda's Candida program!!! There's so much life to live when you don't have to deal with this chronic, unfortunate epidemic!!!

My heart-felt appreciation to Brenda for her wisdom & experience.

–Lumen, Nelson, BC

I just finished the Candida diet (6 weeks). I did very well on it, and feel so, so much better. Although I didn't lose as much weight as I would have liked, I did lose between 10-15 lbs. and just feel so much better. I have a lot more energy, no more hormonal symptoms and I just feel really good. Thanks Brenda for all your great advice and knowledge.

–Deb C, Victoria, BC

SUMMARY

If you have Candida, you need to treat it. The approximate amount of time will be four to six weeks. It is best if you stay on friendly bacteria for a few months afterward. Once you are no longer taking the "Candida Eradicator" product and silver solution, you can move on to the next chapter.

If you do not have Candida, then you are ready to look at the next fast track solution.

CHAPTER 10

Fast Track Solution Five:
Restore Adrenal Balance

There is a great deal of truth to the saying "stress is the root of all our health problems." As you read on, you will clearly see the relationship between stress and your hormones.

Introducing Your Adrenal Glands

First I must introduce you to your adrenal glands. They are two small glands about the size and shape of a flattened prune that sit on top of your kidneys. I refer to your adrenal glands as your "stress glands," because in stressful situations they produce adrenal hormones, along with a myriad of other hormones, to help you deal with stress.

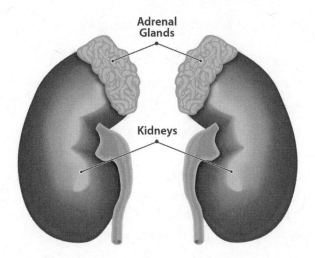

Adrenal
Glands

Kidneys

More Stressors Than You Think

Stress is certainly all of those emotional issues that come up in a day – from parenting your children to driving in rush hour traffic to meeting work deadlines – but you are assaulted by many other types of stressors as well.

Stress can be any burden to your body. This includes emotional, physical, nutritional and chemical sources of stress.

Physical stress comes from things like:

- repetitive strain injuries, such as carpal tunnel syndrome
- back problems
- a burn, any accident, injury or illness
- the stress of chronic pain
- compulsions and addictions
- excessive or incorrect exercise or the opposite – lack of exercise
- headaches
- lack of sleep
- carrying excess weight
- hormonal imbalances
- surgery (this one is an enormous stress on the body)

Chemical stress comes from things like:

- toxins in our personal care products
- dyes and preservatives in our food
- taking recreational or prescription drugs
- smoking
- work environment toxins/fumes in jobs such as hair/beauty salons, drycleaners, automotive shops, painters, plumbers, electricians, welders, janitorial jobs, drywallers, firefighters and delivery drivers, just to name a few

- home environment toxins such as new paint, carpet or furniture fumes, cleaning products and laundry products
- car exhaust

Nutritional stress comes from things like:
- too much alcohol
- junk food
- too much sugar or caffeine
- deficiencies of vitamins, minerals, amino acids and essential fatty acids

Emotional stress comes from things like:
- your current job
- changing or losing your job
- deadlines
- co-workers
- your spouse
- a divorce
- financial worries
- raising children
- looking after aging parents
- death of a friend or family member
- your own retirement or your partner's retirement
- dealing with teenagers
- empty nest syndrome
- going through counseling
- expectations
- selling or buying a house
- renovations
- moving

- dating
- guilt
- worry about anything

All these factors combine together to create ONE HUGE STRESS LOAD in your life.

What Does All This Stress Do?

When the adrenal glands respond to stress, they release hormones such as epinephrine (adrenaline) and norepinephrine (noradrenalin) and cortisol. These stress hormones rally all of your body's resources into "fight or flight" mode by increasing your heart rate and blood pressure, releasing your energy stores for immediate use and sharpening your senses, while shutting down digestion and other secondary functions to conserve energy.

These body responses are useful when physical action is required. Certainly our cave-dwelling ancestors needed this "fight or flight" mode when confronted with an unfriendly saber-toothed tiger. In our modern civilization we no longer have to fight saber-toothed tigers but our bodies are still programmed to respond the same way.

Without any physical outlet, the body reacts to stress by channeling its responses inward to one of the organ systems. You know the feeling of nausea after a fright? It is the feeling you get when your digestive system shuts down under stress. Similarly, extreme tension may shut down your small capillaries in your circulatory system causing things like hypertension, headaches, and fatigue.

Each period of stress should be followed by proper rest and lots of quality nourishment so the adrenals can fully recuperate and rejuvenate to prepare for the next onslaught of stress.

Of course, in today's society most women are constantly maintaining a high level of stress and are not getting enough rest or the proper intake of nutrients.

Eventually this negative combination leads to what I call adrenal fatigue. The adrenals are still functioning, but not optimally, which in turn creates both health and hormonal issues for women of all ages.

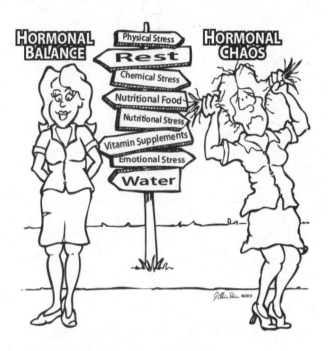

How Stress Causes Hormonal Imbalances

1. Progesterone is the one primary raw material the adrenal glands use for producing the adrenal hormones.

The adrenal glands cannot make cortisol without progesterone. Often referred to as the 'progesterone steal,' your body will steal however much progesterone it needs to make cortisol.

This means the more stress you are under, the more adrenal hormones you produce, and the more progesterone you use up.

Let's walk through this slowly:

Your adrenal glands respond to stress.

Each time you are under stress your adrenals produce adrenal hormones.

Your adrenal glands use progesterone to produce these adrenal hormones.

If you use up progesterone under stress, then estrogen will dominate.

And the more estrogen dominant you are, the more symptoms you will have.

It's starting to make sense, isn't it?

Stress is bad news for any menstruating woman but even worse for women in the perimenopausal phase. I say this because a menstruating woman is still ovulating each month, which means she is producing progesterone every time she ovulates.

Now fast forward in time to perimenopause when you no longer ovulate every month. You are already progesterone deficient (estrogen dominant) by this phase. Then add a lot of stress, and you will use up the very little progesterone you have in order to make your adrenal "stress" hormones.

The combination of not ovulating every month (remember ovulation triggers the release of progesterone from your ovaries) and depleting the existing progesterone because of stress can make the perimenopausal woman very estrogen dominant. This can cause a perimenopausal woman to experience hormonal symptoms she has never had before or can worsen her existing symptoms.

Once you understand how estrogen dominance is very prevalent in the perimenopausal phase, you can easily see why perimenopausal women are so susceptible to hormonal problems such as heavy periods and weight gain around their abdomen, hips and thighs (symptoms of estrogen dominance).

2. Stress leading to excess cortisol production has other negative effects as well. Not only is progesterone used up to make cortisol, progesterone is also the substance from which most of the other steroid hormones are derived, including estrogen and testosterone.

The more progesterone used up under stress, the fewer resources the adrenal glands have to produce the other sex hormones.

This scenario explains one of the reasons that a perimenopausal woman can periodically experience menopausal symptoms. In the perimenopausal stage, there can be times when your ovarian supply of estrogen crashes. Normally your adrenal glands could come to the rescue by producing a backup supply of estrogen. But, if stress has used up all the raw material (progesterone), then a sudden drop in estrogen will result in menopausal symptoms such as hot flashes and/or night sweats.

3. Cortisol and progesterone compete with each other for the same receptor cells. Do you remember the game "musical chairs"? Seven chairs but eight girls – imagine the seven girls are cortisol and the eighth girl is progesterone, and she gets knocked out. Excess cortisol will always beat out progesterone for the receptor cells. Any available progesterone not used for cortisol or other steroid production is at risk of not being utilized properly. This is another way you can become progesterone deficient (estrogen dominant).

4. Adrenal function and thyroid function are intimately related. Approximately 80% of women suffering from adrenal fatigue also experience some form of decreased thyroid function. For these women to get well, the adrenals must be supported first before trying to support thyroid function.

Don't Wait For a Medical Diagnosis

I bet you are wondering why your doctor hasn't diagnosed something as straightforward as adrenal fatigue.

In mainstream medicine, doctors are trained to recognize outright disease, not what we call subclinical illnesses which are conditions that exhibit symptoms but blood work cannot confirm the disorder.

If you let yourself develop Addison's Disease (when the body's cortisol production is severely deficient) or Cushing's Disease (body produces excessively high levels of cortisol), then your doctor can diagnose you. These conditions are the extreme result of serious adrenal imbalance and require immediate medical intervention.

Medical tests can't factor in how you feel. They are designed to determine either a healthy or diseased state in the body. If you want to know whether your adrenal glands are functioning optimally, your symptoms are your best indicator.

WHAT ADRENAL PHASE ARE YOU IN?

Phase One: Balanced Adrenal Function

Barring other health issues, when your adrenal glands are functioning optimally, you should be able to:

- Go to sleep with ease and wake up refreshed
- Have steady energy levels throughout the day
- Adapt to the normal stressors of life
- Experience joyful and happy moods
- Maintain excellent focus, concentration and recall
- Choose salty or sugary food, rather than be a slave to them
- Fight infections and ward off colds and flu
- Rely on a healthy libido
- Get up and go without the need for caffeine
- Be pain free
- Maintain normal blood pressure and water balance

Can you remember this phase? How long has it been? Don't worry (it's another stressor). With the fast track solutions, you can return to (or discover for the first time) this balanced state of being.

Are you in phase one? Yes___ (Bravo! You are a rare gem!) No___

Phase Two: Too Much Cortisol

This phase can be short-lived or go on for a very long time. If you are in this phase, you might not even think there is anything wrong with your life because too much cortisol can initially feel really good.

The upside to cortisol is it raises your energy and focus, but sustained high levels of cortisol will eventually start to take you down.

In the latter part of phase two, you only have to think about "fattening food" and you will increase your belly fat; but try as you might, you just can't lose it.

You also run the risk of developing high blood pressure, insulin resistance (type 2 diabetes), as well as losing focus, concentration and memory.

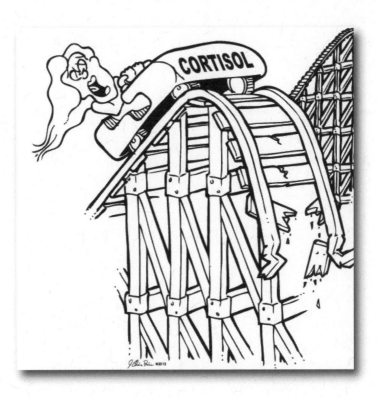

Excess cortisol depletes serotonin (your happy hormone), so over time you will start barking at your spouse and children, become irritable with friends and co-workers, suffer with anxiety and/or depression and have insomnia.

If you are anywhere in phase two, your adrenals are gobbling up your progesterone, and you are starting to get an increasing number of hormonal symptoms as you become more and more estrogen dominant.

If you feel like you are all revved up and can't come down, can't rest, and can't relax, then you are likely riding the cortisol roller coaster and you must get off this ride before you crash and burn!

Is this you? The good news is it's not too late. You can lower your stress and cortisol, drop weight and your blood pressure, regain your memory, and long-lost sex drive, all in addition to feeling happy and calm once again.

Symptoms of too much cortisol are:

- Anxiety and/or panic attacks
- Bone loss
- Fatigue
- High blood pressure
- Hair loss
- Impaired memory
- Insomnia
- Insulin resistance
- Irritability
- Loss of muscle mass
- Low sex drive
- Irregular menstrual cycle, and, sometimes, the cycle can stop altogether
- Mood swings and/or depression
- Tired but wired feeling

- Weight gain at the waist (and after a period of time, limbs look very skinny or slender)

Are you in phase two? Yes____ No____

Phase Three: The Cortisol Flip-Flop

There will be a period of time where your body can flip-flop between producing excess cortisol so you feel like you are in phase two, and not being able to produce enough cortisol so you feel like you are in phase four (adrenal fatigue).

Are you in phase three? Yes____ No____

Phase Four: Adrenal Fatigue

If stress continues without the required rest and nutrients necessary for adrenal rejuvenation, you will eventually end up here. Ninety-nine percent of the women I meet are in phase three or four.

There are many symptoms of adrenal fatigue and some are the same as excess cortisol (phase two); but when your body is not able to produce enough cortisol, you will have difficulties in all of the areas that cortisol influences. You can use the questionnaire below to determine the level of adrenal fatigue that you are currently experiencing. You can also use these symptoms to monitor your recovery.

ADRENAL QUESTIONNAIRE

If you have any of the following symptoms, put the assigned number in the blank. At the end of the questionnaire, add up all your numbers.

To print your own copy of the following adrenal questionnaire visit www.HormoneRollerCoaster.com

2 Low blood pressure or experience dizziness when going from a lying position to a standing position ____

2 A craving for salt or salty foods ___

2 Prone to eczema, hay fever, sneezing attacks, asthma or hives ___

2 Inability to deal with stress ___

2 Tendency to get upset or frustrated easily, quick to cry ___

2 Feeling of being mentally and emotionally overstressed ___

2 Low blood sugar symptoms such as feeling shaky, weak or irritable when hungry, waking up hungry in the night, or feeling your best when eating small amounts of food throughout the day (grazing) ___

2 Chronic pain throughout the body, such as dull aches, joint pains similar to arthritis, and muscle weakness. Sometimes you might even experience pain around the kidneys, sides, and lower back near where the adrenal glands are located ___

2 Food or respiratory allergies ___

2 Bouts of severe infection or recurrent, chronic infections, such as yeast infections ___

2 Inability to tolerate much exercise or you feel worse after exercising ___

2 Depressed and/or moody and/or irritable ___

2 Find it difficult to get going in the morning (not being rested upon awakening) or need caffeine (coffee, tea, and others) to get you going in the morning ___

2 Sweat easily without a temperature increase, or get hot flushes and night sweats ___

2 Tendency to catch colds easily when weather changes ___

2 Weakness prolonged after colds or flu ___

2 Voice rises to a high pitch or gets lost in a stressful situation ___

1 Ridged fingernails ____

1 Sensitivity to exhaust fumes, smoke, smog, and petro-
   chemicals ____

1 Dark circles under your eyes ____

1 Lack of mental alertness or inability to concentrate ____

1 Regular headaches or migraines ____

1 Water retention ____

1 Trouble falling asleep or staying asleep ____

1 Feeling of tiredness all the time ____

1 Low tolerance of loud noises and/or strong odors ____

1 Low tolerance for alcohol, caffeine and other drugs ____

1 Tendency to get a second wind at night ____

1 Haven't felt your best in a long time ____

1 Eyes sensitive to bright light ____

1 Chronic heartburn ____

1 Sweet cravings ____

1 Lack of thirst ____

1 Chronic pain in the lower neck and upper back ____

1 A tightness or lump in your throat that hurts when you are
   emotionally upset ____

1 Form goose bumps easily ____

1 A tendency to startle easily or heart pounds hard from
   unexpected noise ____

   Grand total _____

Pinpointing the level of adrenal fatigue that you are experiencing is not an exact science. You may only have a few symptoms, but they could be so severe that you are still suffering as much adrenal fatigue as someone with many symptoms. The following chart is simply a guide-line to help you determine the condition of your adrenal glands and the amount of adrenal support you will need.

Adrenal Fatigue Guideline

> 0-5 mild fatigue
> 6-22 moderate fatigue
> 23-39 severe fatigue
> 40-54 critically severe fatigue

No matter what condition your adrenal glands are in, there is a solution. I have literally helped hundreds of women return to optimal adrenal function, which of course helped them to restore their health and balance their hormones.

Before we move into solutions, I want to point out that your adrenal glands will be responsible for producing your sex hormones in meno-pause. If you want to avoid the symptoms of menopause, then don't delay. There is no time like the present to ensure your adrenal glands are functioning optimally. You will reap the rewards now and in the future!

SOLUTIONS

Stop the Damage

This is a necessary step for women in all adrenal phases. It is your wake-up call.

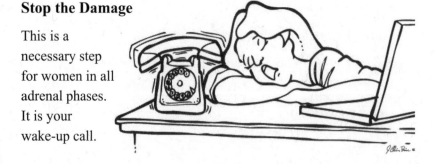

You need to do something about the avalanche of stress!

Any reduction of the stressors in your life will alleviate some of the wear and tear you are putting on your adrenal glands, so you can start the recovery process.

If you are in phase two, you can prevent going into phases three and four by reducing your stressors and lowering your cortisol.

If you are in phase three or four, you must do what you can to reduce the stresses while simultaneously nourishing the adrenal glands.

If you don't minimize your stressors, then you will be continually running up the down escalator.

When I am doing a seminar, women seem to grasp this concept better when I use this following analogy.

The Rewards Are On The Top Floor

Imagine the items you want (health and hormonal balance) are on the top floor of the department store and you have entered the building on the ground level (adrenal fatigue). You look around, and there isn't an escalator going up. The only way to get to the top floor is to run up the down escalator (stress). So you run as hard as you can to get up the down escalator. Even with a lot of effort (equivalent to rest and nutrients), it is going to take a long time to get to the top floor. But what if the down escalator (stress) stopped or slowed down enough so all you had to do was walk up the down escalator stairs? You would certainly get to the rewards (energy, slim body, and happy moods) in a lot less time and with significantly less effort.

What this means is that to rejuvenate your adrenal glands in the least amount of time, with the least amount of effort and cost, you have to reduce the sources of stress so your rejuvenation strategies can work effectively.

It can be hard to minimize emotional stress, I know only too well about all life's stressors.

Brenda Eastwood's Story

At what should have been the most memorable moment in my life, the miracle of adopting a baby girl (I couldn't get pregnant because I was in the final stages of perimenopause at 32), I was trying to win the superwoman award of the century. My (now ex) husband and I returned home from the hospital with a five-day-old baby. After getting up all through the night, I went back to work the next day.

Not only did I continue to get up every night, which is unavoidable with a brand new baby, I continued to make sales calls for my ex-husband and oversee his business. I continued my own nutritional practice, washed cloth diapers, made baby formula from scratch, kept the house clean, did the grocery shopping, cooked the meals and did the laundry. I remember being so tired one Saturday that I put the baby into her wind-up swing and brought it into my bedroom. I cranked up the swing then jumped into bed to sleep for 10 minutes before the swing would stop and my baby would start to fuss, and then repeated the process.

All of the stress was gobbling up my progesterone. No wonder my peri-menopausal symptoms were at an all-time extreme high! The estrogen dominance created such a heavy flow, I was certain I was going to hemorrhage to death. Sometimes I would just sit on the toilet and let the blood pour out. I would soak through tampons or regular pads very quickly, so I used some of my baby's extra cloth diapers as backup pads. I was also getting hot flashes every 20 minutes. Oh, and I shouldn't forget to mention the extreme vaginal dryness. Seriously, I think I actually squeaked when I walked.

Don't let this be you.

Try Adopting These New Habits for Reducing Stress

1. Can you simplify your life? Meaning, are there things (both tangible and not) you can do without? The need to acquire more "things" causes us to work more in order to buy more.

2. Get your kids to pitch in and help carry the load. This is how people managed years ago, even when the majority of women stayed home to look after house and home. It also teaches children responsibility, accountability and appreciation.

3. Say NO more often or at least say "let me get back to you" rather than giving an immediate decision.

4. Figure out what HAS to be done each day and do those tasks first. Then make it a priority to get to bed no later than 11 p.m. whether you are done or not.

5. Get AT LEAST seven hours sleep every night. You can never ever catch up on "lost" sleep, no matter how hard you try.

6. Try co-operative parenting. "I will take your kids to practice this week, if you take my kids next week."

7. Take 10 minutes of quiet time for yourself each day so your mind can rest. This might be used for journaling, reading a book for pleasure, soaking in your tub with candles and relaxing music or simply sitting quietly without doing anything else at all for those 10 precious minutes.

8. What can you take off your plate? Who is putting the pressure on you to do everything you are doing? (The answer is usually YOU!) Since you are the boss of you, be kinder to your most valuable employee.

9. When you make a meal such as soup, stew or casserole, can you make a big batch so there is extra to freeze for another night or to have for lunch the next day?

10. You can't control your boss, or spouse or children, but you can control your chemical and nutritional stressors. I highly recommend putting a bookmark in this spot or at the end of this chapter and going to **Lifestyle Strategies For A Lifetime**, chapters 15 to 22. These chapters will outline the worst chemical and nutritional stressors and give you suggestions on how to minimize their negative impact.

I am sure if you make de-stressing a high priority, you can easily come up with your top 10 choices, such as meditation, either self-guided or using one from a reputable source, activities such as Tai Chi or yoga, more laughter, a regular tea date with your girlfriends, a nice walk in the great outdoors, and the list goes on.

Vacations are great, but have you ever noticed when you return it doesn't take long for you to feel the same way you did before you left? Or, the whole process of the vacation itself proves to be more stressful than it would have been had you stayed home? The de-stressing I am talking about needs to be in the form of daily lifestyle modifications. You cannot expect a two-week annual vacation to compensate for all the stress you put yourself through the other 50 weeks of the year.

LOWER YOUR CORTISOL

Phase Two and Three

You will need to address this issue if you are in phase two or three.

If you are in phase four, there is no cortisol to lower, so you don't need this step.

You might think you need calming herbs because you feel over-whelmed or "stressed out" very easily. But this is typical and common for anyone with any amount of adrenal fatigue. You won't handle stress well because your adrenals are too tired to produce your "stress hor-mones," leaving you feeling challenged by stressful situations which causes more stress to your adrenal glands causing them to become even more tired.

If you are in phase four, the best area for you to focus on is feeding your adrenal glands with specific restorative nutrients (discussed later in this chapter). The more nourished the adrenals become, the better you are able to cope with and adapt to stress.

There Is Always An Exception To The Rule: Phase Four

If you are exclusively in phase four and yet you feel better taking a cortisol lowering herb, continue to take it. If your symptoms worsen, then you don't need this kind of support.

Drugs force a reaction in the body, whereas nutrients and herbs work gently to support your body and its functions. The beauty of my recommendations is there is no harm in trying the herbs I am going to suggest.

Go with your gut. Pay attention to how you feel when you take them and you will know if they are right for you or not.

My Top Two Cortisol Lowering Choices

There are many herbs to choose from. For example, everywhere you turn there is an article promoting the benefits of Rhodiola for stress. I have heard testimonials from people who have benefited from it, but I have never suggested it to my clients because the wrong dosage can cause anxiety and the "jitters." Rhodiola can have a stimulating effect at lower amounts and a sedating effect at higher amounts. It can be difficult to find the right dosage for each person.

If you are taking Rhodiola right now and you feel it is working for you, then keep taking it. If you haven't tried it yet, I would opt for one of the other choices I am about to give you.

1. Holy Basil

Holy basil has stood the test of time. Being used in India for thousands of years for its medicinal properties, it is an adaptogen, meaning it brings balance to the entire body. This herb works very well for reducing depression, stress and anxiety.

Holy Basil improves memory, and reduces unclear thinking and mental fog. It balances the hormones and helps reduce excess cortisol levels. It has anti-inflammatory properties and is helpful in maintaining normal blood sugar levels as well.

The dosage will depend on the strength and quality of the product you purchase.

The one I have been recommending is 500 mg per capsule. You might need to experiment to find the best dosage and time of day for you.

It would be nice to have a crystal ball to figure this out for you, but this is part of the process: becoming educated and learning to pay attention to your body so you know what it needs.

Here are some suggestions to try.

    1 in the morning and 1 after lunch

    1 in the morning and 1 mid-afternoon

    2 in the morning and 1 at lunch or mid-afternoon

    2 in the morning

    2 in the mid-afternoon

I do not suggest taking it later than three p.m. as it has the possibility of interrupting sleep in some circumstances. Holy Basil is not intended for long-term use. When you are no longer feeling "wired," stop taking it. You can take it again if you need it, or you can take it sporadically on an as-needed basis.

What My Clients Have to Say About Holy Basil

I take two Holy Basil in the morning and it seems to keep me calm during the day. Thanks again!!

        –Denise G, Calgary, Alta

Things are looking good. Perhaps Holy Basil is my answer! My "issues" are really improving!! Anxiety is really low, my mood is great, and I am sleeping really well. - YEY!!!

        –Linda I, Victoria, BC

2. Passionflower

Don't let the name fool you, Passionflower is not the aphrodisiac you might be seeking. This herb has been traditionally used for calming.

It is potent enough for an adult, yet safe enough to give to a child.

Again, the dosage will depend on the strength and quality of the product you purchase. The one I have been recommending for years is a liquid tincture.

Suggested Usage: Start with 15 drops two to three times per day and increase to a max of $1^1/_2$ teaspoons four times per day if needed for more calming action. It is a safe herb, so feel free to experiment and discover what works best for you.

Passionflower can be taken before bed (as opposed to Holy Basil which should not be taken before bed). In fact, taken before bed, Passion-flower can be a soothing sleep-aid.

If poor sleep is a problem for you, don't wait to take Passionflower just before bed, because it is usually the accumulated stress and tension of the day keeping you awake at night. If you are a poor sleeper, I suggest taking some during the day as well as at bedtime. Passionflower can be safely combined with GABA (see next page) and/or magnesium and/or Holy Basil (although Holy Basil should not be taken in the evening).

What My Clients Have to Say About Passionflower

I will be getting rid of a good deal of stress very soon so that should help. In the interim, taking Passionflower throughout the day helps.

–Joni C, Calgary, Alta

Thank you. I have been taking Passionflower and have had no interruptions with my sleep except when the cat crashes into my bed-room door in the early hours of the morning. Thanks again Brenda, you are a genius.

–Valerie A, Victoria, BC

Something For <u>All</u> Adrenal Phases

3. GABA: Nature's Stress Buster

GABA (gamma-aminobutyric acid) is your brain's natural Valium. Actually Valium is one of many tranquilizers designed to mimic or amplify GABA's naturally calming effects.

Taken as a supplement, GABA can not only help you turn off stress reactions after an upset, it can actually help prevent a stressful response when taken prior to an expected ordeal (such as before an exam or getting on an airplane).

It can also be used to reduce what I call "busy brain" and anxiety. (Note: anxiety is often a secondary symptom of low moods or depression. If you have anxiety, refer to the e-manual "The Natural Way to Great Moods and Happiness" found at www.HormoneRollerCoaster.com). I also highly recommend the book *The Mood Cure* by Julia Ross, M.A.

GABA will work almost immediately, so you can take it periodically as you need to in specific situations, or you can take it daily to build up your own natural stores again. There is no "hangover" or groggy feeling when using GABA and there are no negative side effects if you abruptly stop taking it.

You will not feel drugged when taking GABA, but you should feel something in the way of an overall calming sensation or ability to focus on the task at hand without distraction. It should not make you drowsy or unable to function as a drug might. If it does not appear to be helping, then it isn't what you need, and I would suggest trying Passionflower instead. Or if GABA alone isn't enough, you can combine it with Passionflower and/or Holy Basil and/or magnesium.

If you need fast action for an anxiety attack, you can dump the contents of a GABA capsule under your tongue. It doesn't taste great but it will usually start to work in less than five minutes.

<u>Suggested use</u>: Start with the lesser dosage listed and increase gradually only if you need more calming action. The longer you take GABA, the less you will need.

The GABA I have been recommending for years has 500 mg per capsule.

For anxiety take 1 to 3 capsules mid-morning – approximately two hours after your breakfast, and then take 1 to 3 capsules approximately two hours after your lunch. Because it is an amino acid (which competes with other amino acids from protein foods), you will get a better response if you take GABA on an empty stomach or away from food, but it will still work if you have food in your stomach.

If you don't sleep well, you can take 1 to 3 capsules mid-evening and then 1 to 3 capsules before bed. If you wake up with "busy brain," you can take 1 to 3 capsules to help you go back to sleep.

You can also use different combinations; for example, you may find 1 capsule mid-evening is calming, but you need 3 capsules before bed to help you fall asleep. Keep in mind GABA is not a sleep aid but its calming action in the brain allows your body to go through its natural processes to fall asleep much more easily.

Possible side effects: The only noted side effect is some people will get what feels like a niacin rush if they take too many at one time. This prickly heat sensation will subside in about 30 minutes. This may feel like anxiety or a hot flash, along with an elevated heart rate. Should you experience this, relax. It will pass and next time you take GABA, take 1 capsule less.

I Love GABA and So Do My Clients!

I love GABA. The anxiety came along with the aldosteronism and the GABA was my life saver. The Dr. wanted to give me an anti depressant and I said no thank you, I'll handle this myself which I did with the GABA and exercise. It is much better now and I always keep the GABA close by. I can't imagine where I would be if Sue hadn't introduced me to you and the Inner Circle. Thank you for everything you do. Everything I have come to you for has worked beautifully. Thanks again for ALL your help.

–Juanita C, Vancouver, BC

Thanks Brenda.....I took one GABA before bed last night and DID NOT WAKE UP ONCE!!! You are my angel and I am so grateful you came into my life.

–Christa M, Fernie, BC

My dad just finished yet another round of radiation. He's hanging in there, but it is difficult for all concerned right now.

As for me, I'm surviving because of the Daily Essential Nutrients, magnesium and GABA! They are REALLY helping!

–Catherine S, Cochrane, Alta

I would like to place an order for 3 bottles of GABA please. I've been working 9 shifts per week for a month now and have been taking this product about 4 mornings per week and it's amazing. My stress levels should be extremely high but I'm not stressed at all. Wow! I knew it worked but I didn't have an opportunity to try it with an ongoing stress load until now. Thanks.

–Carole M, Langford, BC

I kept meaning to email you and thank you for letting me know about GABA. As my story goes, a couple of years ago, I started getting what I call "anxiety" attacks, a "rush" throughout my body.

The Dr. of course gave me tranquilizers, but I never did take one, but every morning this was the first thing on my mind, I was getting very anxious just thinking today was the day I would not be able to control the attack!! (As I would try and calm myself down during each attack) I was getting up to 3 a day, anytime and anywhere!! I use to wonder if I was going to have to live with this for the next 30 years :-(But now I take 2 GABA in the morning, and I have not felt better!! I have not had ANY attacks, and my fist thoughts in the morning are "what a great day it is!!" Anyway a BIG THANKS BRENDA. Without you many, many people would be living a sad life!!!

–Kim B, Nanaimo, BC

I just adore the GABA. I am a woman of steel now! My mind might have a fear thought yet my body remains placid. It is a miracle.

–Alice B, Vancouver, BC

I keep a bottle beside my bed and if I am having trouble drifting off to sleep because of busy brain, then I take one and in 20 minutes I am asleep.

–Brenda Eastwood, Victoria, BC

NUTRIENTS FOR REJUVENATING YOUR ADRENAL GLANDS

Exciting news! You have already begun the process of adrenal rejuvenation with the nutrients you have been taking as part of the **Fast Track Foundation**.

Vitamins like C, E and all the B vitamins (especially pantothenic acid) have crucial roles in the production and actions of stress hormones. And magnesium provides necessary energy not only for your adrenals, but for every cell in your body to function properly. Calcium and several trace minerals, like zinc, manganese, selenium, and iodine, provide calming effects in the body. These minerals can help relieve the stress associated with adrenal fatigue and imbalance, which will ultimately restore normal cortisol output.

Even though there are some key nutrients which are critical for adrenal gland recovery, it is important to realize your adrenal glands need an entire broad spectrum of vitamins, minerals, essential fatty acids, antioxidants and amino acids to function properly.

If the adrenal glands are missing any of these nutrients, they cannot produce adequate amounts of adrenal hormones. A deficiency of any one of the required nutrients can cause a breakdown in the manufacturing process.

The beauty of the Daily Essential Nutrients and magnesium citrate is they are the foundational nutrients your adrenals need to recover.

Women in phase one and phase two with minimal stress should only require the nutrients in the **Fast Track Foundation** to keep their adrenal glands in optimal health.

Women in phase three and four will need to supplement with some additional targeted nutrients over and above the **Fast Track Foundation**.

How To Select Additional Adrenal Support

Entire books have been dedicated to the topic of adrenal fatigue, which is why I cannot possibly cover all the intricacies of adrenal rejuvenation within the context of this book.

What I can offer however, is my clinical experience dating back to 1981, thus providing you with the absolute most proven methods of restoring your adrenal glands. If you follow the steps I have outlined, you will experience the health and hormonal balance that is possible with optimal adrenal function.

The operative words are "if you follow."

You can't purchase supplements and hope they will magically work by looking at them. You also can't expect to get results by only half-heartedly following the directions.

It is scientifically proven;
vitamins that sit on the shelf don't work

Perhaps "can't" is not the right word. My husband has this saying, "do whatever you like because you will anyway," and it's true that you can absolutely do whatever you like and you probably will.

But think about it. How much sense does it make to pay good money for advice and supplements, then not follow through? It would be like hiring an accountant to do your tax return and not submitting it. Or paying for an expensive membership fee at the gym for a whole year and only showing up for the first month. Or getting a prescription from your doctor and only taking half the dosage.

Balancing your hormones is simple, but it isn't easy. You have to put in time and effort. If you want results, take action and follow through. I promise the rewards will be worth it.

There are many types of adrenal support. To fully rejuvenate your adrenal glands, you may need one or a combination.

The following section will outline three of my most successful options and give you step-by-step directions on selecting and using additional nutritional support for fully rejuvenating your adrenal glands.

There are three categories:

    1. Vitamin Therapy

    2. Herbal Therapy

    3. Glandular Therapy

1. Vitamin Therapy for Adrenal Support

If appropriate, the next step is to add pantothenic acid. Pantothenic acid is also known as vitamin B5. As it is part of the entire B complex, it is present in any multi B complex.

However, in order to effectively support your adrenal glands, it is needed in much higher doses than what is provided in the Daily Essential Nutrients.

If you have two or more of the following symptoms, I would definitely add pantothenic acid (vitamin B5) as a targeted nutrient to help repair your adrenal glands.

Typical Symptoms of a Pantothenic Acid Deficiency:

____ Fatigue

____ Irritability

___ Listlessness, nervousness

___ Poor appetite

___ Depression

___ Digestive disturbances

___ Quarrelsomeness

___ Headaches

___ Increased need for sleep

___ Recurrent respiratory infections

To do proper vitamin therapy for the adrenal glands, you need trace minerals, B complex, the correct form of vitamin C (all of which are in your Daily Essential Nutrients) and higher doses of pantothenic acid. Instead of just taking your Daily Essential Nutrients in the morning, take it after both breakfast and lunch, along with 1,000 mg of pantothenic acid (B5).

Most people with adrenal fatigue are deficient in pantothenic acid; however, if you do not have at least two of the pantothenic acid symptoms listed above, do not take this additional supplement. Instead go on to the herbal therapy.

If you decide to add the pantothenic acid, start with that and monitor your results before determining if you need any further adrenal support; or if you are suffering with extreme adrenal fatigue, you may wish to add another adrenal support right away.

For recommendations on pantothenic acid (vitamin B5), B complex and buffered vitamin C go to www.HormoneRollerCoaster.com

YOUR PROGRAM WITH PANTHOTHENIC ACID
FOR ADRENAL SUPPORT

After Breakfast:
Daily Essential Nutrients
1,000 mg of pantothenic acid
200 mg of B6 (from ovulation to period) **and/or** I-3-C

After Lunch:
(or after dinner as long as you don't get too energized and can't sleep)
Daily Essential Nutrients
1,000 mg of pantothenic acid
I-3-C

Before Bed:
400 to 700 mg elemental magnesium from magnesium citrate

BARE BONES ADRENAL SUPPORT

If you don't want to repeat the entire Daily Essentials a second time of the day, you can do this.

After Breakfast:
Daily Essential Nutrients
1,000 mg of pantothenic acid
200 mg of B6 (from ovulation to period) **and/or** I-3-C

After Lunch:
(or after dinner as long as you don't get too energized and can't sleep)
1 B complex
1,000 mg of buffered vitamin C
1,000 mg of pantothenic acid
I-3-C

Before Bed:
400 to 700 mg elemental magnesium from magnesium citrate

2. Herbal Therapy for Adrenal Support

Please read all three choices first before deciding which one best suits your needs.

Choice A: Wild Yam

Wild yam has been used for decades to assist people with adrenal fatigue. It is a hormone balancer with antispasmodic properties, making it a great choice for abdominal cramps, bowel spasms and menstrual cramps. Wild Yam is also known for its ability to soothe nerves.

Overall, it is the most effective herb for women of all ages. It helps menopausal women with hot flashes and night sweats, and it helps women in their menstruating years with PMS and menstrual cramps. This is why it also makes it a perfect choice for perimenopausal women who get both PMS and menopausal symptoms.

Suggested Use: The dosage will depend on the strength and quality of the product you purchase.

The one I have been recommending is 500 mg per capsule. You might need to experiment a bit to find the best dosage and time of day for you.

To start, try 1 capsule twice a day. If you don't notice any improvement in your adrenal symptoms after two weeks, you can try 2 capsules twice a day. If you don't notice any improvement in your adrenal symptoms after an additional two weeks at this dosage, then you will need to try another remedy for supporting your adrenal glands. Very occasionally women will have an opposite reaction to too much Wild Yam, whereby it will worsen their symptoms or cause them to have hot flashes and night sweats. If this happens to you, cut back on your dosage or switch to another herb.

What My Clients Have to Say About Wild Yam

I took your advice and added Wild Yam to my regime and WOW what a difference it has made to my life. I noticed an incredible increase in energy almost right away. The perimenopausal symptoms of night sweats, mood swings and hot flashes I had been experiencing have gone. I feel great. Thank you Brenda! I will continue to tell my friends about your website. Thank you again.

–Gail T, Victoria, BC

*I have to say I'm delighted with the extra energy the Wild Yam Capsules are giving me. Bonus... I've lost 10 pounds following your **Lifestyle Strategies for a Lifetime**. Thanks!*

–Terry P, Vancouver, BC

(Note: She is referring to **Lifestyle Strategies For A Lifetime,** chapters 15 to 22).

I cannot believe the results I am having from attending your workshop. I have been taking Wild Yam Herb since October 26 and I can't tell you how awesome I feel. I have no PMS symptoms at all and had a virtually no cramping at that time of the month. I wish I had known about wild yam years ago. Any of you out there suffering, get on this herb. Thanks a million.

–Karen M, Nanaimo, BC

I want to thank you for introducing me to your knowledge, experience and awareness of what I can do for my body. I have not felt this good for many years. I noticed a difference in energy within 36 hours of starting with Wild Yam.

–Marlene B, Nanaimo, BC

Just a quick note to say how enjoyable the seminar was and how your fun attitude kept everyone interested. I have been taking the wild yam capsules & sleeping much better.

–Harbans J, Parksville, BC

Choice B: Suma (Brazilian Ginseng)

This can be a great choice if you are in phase four and don't have any menstrual cramps. I do not usually advise it for phase three because it does provide energy, and women in phase three are usually already feeling wired from the excess cortisol.

Suma is an adaptogen herb because it helps the body adapt to many types of stresses. Suma helps to restore sexual function. Because Suma can stimulate the production of estrogen only if the body needs it, Suma is a great adrenal supplement for perimenopausal women who are getting occasional hot flashes and or night sweats.

Suggested Use: The dosage will depend on the strength and quality of the product you purchase.

The one I have been recommending is 520 mg per capsule. You might need to experiment a bit to find the best dosage for you.

Take 1 capsule twice a day (with or without food). Some women are really sensitive to Suma and can only take 1 capsule in the morning; if they take another one later in the evening, they are too energized and can't sleep. Some women's adrenals are so fatigued, they do best with 2 capsules twice a day.

Start with 1 capsule twice a day and adjust up or down. You may find 2 capsules in the morning and none later in the day or 2 capsules in the morning and 1 later in the day may work best for you. Maximum dosage is 2 capsules twice a day.

What My Clients Have to Say About Suma

Just wanted you to know I ran out of Suma and I wasn't going to replace it - but the old me is back and she isn't interested. If I don't go back on the Suma the chances of me getting pregnant will be pretty slim so I will definitely be ordering today!

–Charlene M, Vancouver, BC

Just want to let you know the Suma has been wonderful - lots of energy for everything including sex!

–Judy F, Victoria, BC

Once again I want to thank you for getting my life back on track. I have never felt better. I even have my mom trying out the Daily Essential Nutrients. I attended your workshop back on March 7 in Calgary. It was an "aha" moment for me. I was becoming more depressed each year, especially in Jan. and Feb. I needed to get myself feeling better or my Doctor was going to put me on anti-depressants. By Thursday after the Sat. workshop, I was definitely feeling better. I am taking the Daily Essential Nutrients and Suma after breakfast and then Suma, and Magnesium in the evening. Thank you.

–Cindy H, Calgary, Alta

Thank you so much for recommending I add Suma to my daily regime. I have noticed more energy and in increase in my sex drive. In fact, within a few weeks I was even attracted to my own husband again *grin ...HE thanks you!

–Meg B, Victoria, BC

Choice C: Licorice

This is an herb and not the sweet licorice you buy to eat. Licorice is helpful for normalizing ovulation in women experiencing infrequent menstruation. It stimulates and sustains adrenal function without depleting it. It helps to raise blood sugar levels to normal. Licorice also has mild laxative properties.

I have observed that women who crave black licorice do well with this herb (no, eating licorice will not help). Also it is a good choice for women with low blood pressure or those trying to get pregnant or those who know they are not ovulating regularly.

Suggested use: The dosage will depend on the strength and quality of the product you purchase.

The one I have been recommending is 470 mg per capsule. You might need to experiment a bit to find the best dosage for you.

Start with 1 capsule twice a day (with or without food). You can increase to 2 in the morning and 1 in the evening if you aren't noticing any improvement in your adrenal symptoms. The maximum recommended dosage is 2 capsules twice a day. (Note: Licorice is not meant to be used long-term. Use for a maximum of three months or alternate with other herbs.)

Helpful Tips

Many herbs can lose their effectiveness over time, so to maintain the benefits of any herb, rotate it with another herb or stop taking it for a couple of weeks every four to six months. Licorice should be rotated more often and not used for more than three months consecutively.

Always return to the product and/or dosage that was working for you, if you happen to experience a worsening of symptoms by reducing the dosage or stopping the product.

Following are some examples of how your program could look.

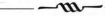

ADRENAL SUPPORT PROGRAM EXAMPLES

Example A

After Breakfast:
    Daily Essential Nutrients
    1,000 mg of pantothenic acid
    200 mg of B6 (from ovulation to period) **and/or** I-3-C
    Wild yam **and/or** suma **and/or** licorice

After Lunch:
(or after dinner as long as you don't get too energized and can't sleep)
    Daily Essential Nutrients
    1,000 mg of pantothenic acid
    Wild yam **and/or** suma **and/or** licorice
    I-3-C

Before Bed:
    400 to 700 mg elemental magnesium from magnesium citrate

Example B

After Breakfast:
    Daily Essential Nutrients
    1,000 mg of pantothenic acid
    200 mg of B6 (from ovulation to period) **and/or** I-3-C
    Wild yam **and/or** suma **and/or** licorice

After Lunch:
(or after dinner as long as you don't get too energized and can't sleep)
    1 B complex
    1,000 mg of buffered vitamin C
    1,000 mg of pantothenic acid
    I-3-C
    Wild yam **and/or** suma **and/or** licorice

Before Bed:
    400 to 700 mg elemental magnesium from magnesium citrate

Example C

After Breakfast:
    Daily Essential Nutrients
    200 mg of B6 (from ovulation to period) **and/or** I-3-C
    Wild yam **and/or** suma **and/or** licorice

After Lunch or Dinner:
    I-3-C
    Wild yam **and/or** suma **and/or** licorice

Before Bed:
    400 to 700 mg elemental magnesium from magnesium citrate

3. Glandular Therapy for Adrenal Support

Glandular therapy can be added to your vitamin therapy and/or your herbal support. I don't recommend skipping directly to the glandular support because I believe the success of any adrenal program stems first from the correct balance of nutrients and herbal support. The best results can be expected when glandular therapy has been used in conjunction with or following my recommended vitamin and/or herbal therapies.

Adrenal Concentrate

Glandular concentrates are made by removing water, fiber and fat from organs and glands of animals, usually cattle or sheep. The remaining dry tissue is concentrated and pressed into tablets. Nutritional glandular supplements are not hormones, do not contain hormones and do not act as hormones.

I never would have believed taking a glandular concentrate would help, but it does. I can't explain it beyond the theory of "like cells help like cells." Cells in our bodies die at the rate of several million per hour. Whenever new cells are required, the DNA (chemical blueprint) sends out RNA (messenger chemical) to gather the necessary materials; and if you are taking an adrenal concentrate supplement, then the RNA can gather those specific materials to rebuild your adrenal cells.

The only person who should not take an adrenal concentrate is a vegan. Anyone else can add this adrenal support at any time in their adrenal recovery program.

Suggested Use: Adrenal concentrate formulas differ hugely from brand to brand, so it always best to simply follow the dosage on the label. If you notice a worsening of symptoms while taking a glandular product, discontinue immediately.

My Suggested Nutritional Products

You will find my suggested nutritional products at:
www.HormoneRollerCoaster.com

TYPICAL MISTAKES WOMEN MAKE WHEN REJUVENATING THEIR ADRENAL GLANDS

1. Quitting Adrenal Support Too Soon

Ideally, you should start seeing improvements in your adrenal fatigue symptoms within 30 days, and some women see them sooner. When you start feeling better, do not quit your adrenal support. That would be like quitting the gym the second you see any muscle definition or weight loss.

Don't let your adrenals fool you. Just because you are feeling better, doesn't mean they are fully rejuvenated.

It will take a MINIMUM OF 90 DAYS to completely rejuvenate your adrenal glands

It could take as long as a year to recover. It could take even longer if you have years of accumulated stress or still live a high-stress lifestyle. It might never happen at all if you ignore the wake up call to de-stress your life. Some women continue to ride this roller coaster of some adrenal repair followed by another burn out. They never reduce their stressors and/or don't stay with their adrenal support program long enough to experience life with optimal adrenal function.

Women who are totally burned out or who have post traumatic stress disorder (PTSD), could potentially need to be on the adrenal rejuvenation program for as long as two to five years.

The amount of time you need to be on adrenal support will depend on your current level of adrenal fatigue and the amount of stressors in your life.

2. Not Giving Enough Support

If you have experienced a lot of stress, not only will you need to be on adrenal support longer, you will most likely need a combination of adrenal therapies all at one time.

3. Not Returning to Adrenal Support During Stressful Times

One of my clients used to keep a bottle of pantothenic acid (vitamin B5) in her cupboard to add to her **Fast Track Foundation** every time her mother-in-law came for a visit. This may be what you need during tax season, through a busy time at work, if you decide to take on a huge project or if you find yourself in one of the many emotional stress situations listed earlier in this chapter.

If you are going through a particularly stressful time, remember to take care of yourself by taking your preferred adrenal therapy. Don't wait until you are suffering with adrenal fatigue again before adding your adrenal therapies. It's easier to support your body through the stressful time than to try and fix it after the damage is done.

4. Expecting Your Supplements to Do All the Work

It would be nice if all you had to do was pop a few supplements, but it doesn't quite work that way. You must do what you can to alleviate the stresses in your life; otherwise you will be constantly running up a down escalator.

Remember, you might not have control over your boss or your children or your job, but you can control some of your lifestyle choices. If you haven't done so already, this is a good time to put a bookmark in this spot and go to **Lifestyle Strategies For A Lifetime**, chapters 15 to 22, so you can learn ways to alleviate some of your nutritional and chemical stress.

5. Adding More To Do When You Feel Better

I am not helping you rejuvenate your adrenal glands so you can take on more stress! If you do this, you will only wear out your adrenal glands again and again.

6. Discounting Your Situation

Women discount the possibility of adrenal fatigue because they just "do what they do," which is a lot! Most women have a full plate. They are juggling their jobs, or furthering their education, volunteering, homeschooling, raising a family, looking after the house, maintaining a garden, caring for aging parents and helping out a friend in need. Maybe it's because they don't slow down long enough to think about how they truly feel, let alone allow themselves some rest and downtime. Have you ever noticed women are always looking after everyone else first?

I am astounded by what we women can do, but putting one foot in front of the other because we need to does not mean we aren't tired, stressed and in desperate need of adrenal support (as well as other types of support).

7. Forcing Yourself to Exercise

Exercise can give you a boost, but if you are pushing yourself to exercise and then feel worse afterwards, then you don't have enough juice in your batteries right now to push that hard. If you have severe adrenal fatigue, you may need to cut back on your exercise program to conserve your energy and allow your adrenals to heal. When you are feeling better, you can begin to slowly ramp up your exercise program again.

SUMMARY

Your adrenal glands are your stress glands because they support you in responding to stress. The more stress in your life, the more worn out your adrenal glands get.

Adrenal imbalance leads to an entire cascade of issues and symptoms.

1. Estrogen dominance (sore breasts, heavy periods, depression, headaches, etc)

2. Adrenal fatigue (fatigue, inability to handle stress well, mood swings, hot flashes, night sweats, low blood sugar, arthritic pain and more).

3. Thyroid dysfunction (unjustified weight gain and/or difficulty losing weight; constipation; heavier, more frequent and more painful periods; hair loss; muscle cramps; water retention, etc)

Stress can be emotional (the one everyone relates to), chemical (i.e. the toxins you absorb through skin care products), physical (i.e. chronic pain) and nutritional (i.e. eating processed food). No wonder women's adrenal glands are in such bad shape!

I rarely meet a woman who doesn't need adrenal support. The best way to decide whether you need adrenal support or not is to review your stress history and answer the adrenal questions. And the only way to recover is to take ACTION.

$$Time + Effort = Results$$

If you are currently on the Candida program, please wait until you have concluded it before proceeding to adrenal rejuvenation.

If you don't need to rejuvenate your adrenal glands, please proceed to the next chapter.

If you are ready to take action and help your adrenal glands recover so they can function optimally, and if you haven't done so already, please put a bookmark in this spot and go now to **Lifestyle Strategies For A Lifetime**, chapters 15 to 22.

Adrenal Rejuvenation Testimonials

I'd like to postpone our appointment. Since I began taking your recommended adrenal support supplements last month, along with the kelp you also suggested, I have been feeling so good I cannot even remember what I wanted to talk to you about. All my perimenopausal symptoms are gone. I am sleeping wonderfully, I have energy, and my mood is great. I am feeling optimistic and I am releasing unnecessary weight - at long last!! So, if you don't mind I'd like to continue on with these supplements and see where this all goes.

Thanks - as usual you have given me back my healthy life!!! You are amazing!

–Denise G, Calgary, Alta

I think I am a walking example of adrenal support therapy and recovery. I have done it all at one time or another and through trial and error have found what works best for me. I can't believe how much better I feel from 4 years ago! Now I know my body well enough to read the signs of when I need to add certain supplements to keep me going or get me back on my feet again. I can't thank you enough. I hope there are many, many more women that will be thanking you like I have in the future!

–Megan B, Victoria, BC

"There's a need for
accepting responsibility -
for a person's life and
making choices that are not
just ones for immediate
short-term comfort.
You need to make an
investment, and the
investment is in health
and education."

~Buzz Aldrin

CHAPTER 11

Fast Track Solution Six:
Ensure Proper Bowel Function

Wait!! Don't skip over this chapter.

F rom all my years of experience, I know most women don't think they have improper bowel function. How would you know? It isn't usually a hot topic of conversation over coffee. I can assure you that eliminating one pencil thin stool, a smattering of rabbit pellets or a massive cow pie every day is not proper bowel function. Eliminating every other day or once a week is not regular either!

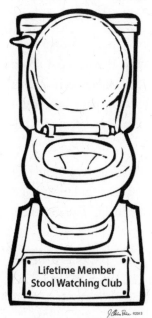

**Lifetime Member
Stool Watching Club**

So what is proper bowel function and what does it have to do with your hormonal balance?

Before we begin you will need to join an elite club. I founded this small, local club years ago and now it has thousands of international members. It is free to join although initiation may cause you some squeamishness; but, for full health value, membership is a requirement.

It is called "The Stool Watching Club." To become a member, you will need to memorize the following rules of proper bowel function.

Proper Bowel Function:

- Every person should have at least two to three bowel movements per day (one per meal). One movement does not necessarily have to follow each meal, you just need to eliminate two to three times per day.

- There should be no stress or straining during a bowel movement.

- The total stool length per movement should measure from the crease of your wrist to the bend of your elbow.

- The diameter should be the size of the circle you make by placing your pointer finger at the bend in your thumb.

- The stool should be light to medium brown in color, free of undigested food, non-odorous, and mostly floating.

Note: the words "bowel" and "colon" are interchangeable.

Without proper bowel function, the food remnants and its digestive components you should be eliminating stay in your body to rot and decay. This rotting fecal material produces the most toxic chemicals known to mankind.

Improper elimination leaves a gluey residue along your intestinal wall, which accumulates day after day, year after year. Because the colon has relatively few nerve endings, it can withstand this accumulation without registering pain. Therefore, in the absence of pain or outright colon disease, without knowing it, you might have a problem relating to your colon.

The toxic gases produced from the rotting fecal material can get trapped and cause most of the problems that are usually labeled and grouped together under the heading of indigestion including flatulence, burping, heartburn, and bloating.

Your intestines are designed to absorb nutrients; so along with the nutrients, when there is rotting fecal matter trapped, you also absorb the toxins into your bloodstream. Since your blood feeds the cells of your body, your blood then delivers these toxins to your cells, which can create a whole host of ailments anywhere in your body – from acne to headaches.

Toxins releasing through your skin can cause issues such as psoriasis and profuse sweating, and the smell of rotting fecal matter creates bad breath, body and/or foot odor.

Many organs reside in close proximity to each other within the small confines of your body trunk. As fecal material accumulates to a weight of anywhere from 5 to 40 pounds, the colon expands and can exert pressure on neighboring organs or tissues, creating problems such as varicose veins, weak bladder and pain at ovulation.

The buildup of fecal material lining your intestines can inhibit nutrient absorption from both the foods you eat and the natural supplements you ingest.

This waste can collect to form what looks like a clogged drain or it can bulge outward, stretching the intestinal lining, causing a balloon-like appearance, which can then show up as a bloated or protruding abdomen. A clogged colon interferes with the weight loss process. If you want to lose excess weight, you must clean your colon.

The stretched intestinal lining loses all elasticity making it even more difficult to achieve proper elimination. This is why some women can-not improve their elimination no matter what positive lifestyle changes they make.

Our major eliminating organs are our colon, lungs, kidney and skin. These organs are responsible for keeping our body cleansed and nourished through regular elimination of waste and foreign material.

When any of these eliminative channels is overburdened and/or over-worked, then the other organs need to work overtime to dispose of the excess debris and toxins. This is how someone who is not eliminating properly via their bowels could end up with chronic sinus or lung congestion.

Poor elimination is associated with outright colon problems such as diverticulitis and irritable bowel syndrome (IBS).

Habitual constipation leaves toxic residues adhering to the intestinal lining. These toxic substances can lead to irritation and inflammation known as colitis.

And, last but not least – the most important reason to ensure proper bowel function is your colon excretes the hormones you no longer need. A clogged colon leads to ESTROGEN DOMINANCE!

THE CONNECTION TO YOUR HORMONES

1. If you cannot properly eliminate the estrogen via your bowel, then you will reabsorb it back into your circulation.

2. Every minute of every day, about two quarts of blood pass through the liver. When the liver is functioning at full capacity, it can filter about 99% of the toxins out of your blood before it is sent back through the body. The liver filters out the toxins that have entered your body through digestion, skin and the respiratory system.

If you are not eliminating properly, the toxins from your bowel are absorbed into your bloodstream and must be filtered through your liver. This adds an extra stress to the liver, which is already struggling with a toxic load from over 50,000 chemicals that have been introduced to our daily living since World War II.

Over time this toxic load can lead to slight liver dysfunction, whereby the liver is unable to do all of its jobs optimally. The liver is responsible for over 500 functions in your body. One of the huge roles your liver plays is to break down hormones after they have served their messenger function to their target cells.

This means a healthy functioning liver will "dispose" of estrogen after it has been used. If the liver does not metabolize estrogen properly, estrogen dominance can result.

You see why I have included either B6 and/or I-3-C in the **Fast Track Foundation**. Both nutrients help the liver excrete excess estrogen.

But the root of the problem can begin in the colon. One of the liver's jobs is to break down estrogen and dump it into your colon for elimination. Therefore you need to maintain proper bowel function so:

a. You can eliminate your excess estrogen.

b. There is no toxic waste in the colon to burden the liver.

BRENDA EASTWOOD'S STORY

My first experience with bowel health was both painful and embarrassing. I was getting very severe lower abdominal pains. When I could no longer work because I was doubled over with pain, I finally went to see my doctor.

Now, you would think by the age of 19 not only would I have heard the word "bowel," I would actually know what it meant. But I didn't.

During the examination, my doctor asked, "How often do you have a bowel movement?" I looked at him with this deadpan stare. Of course I didn't answer; I couldn't answer. I had no idea what he was asking me. He finally realized I was clueless and he turned a bright shade of red before rephrasing the question to "How often do you poop?"

Oh, now I turned a bright red and still couldn't answer him because I had no idea how often I pooped or didn't poop. It wasn't something I was in the habit of tracking (how times have changed!). I wanted to shrink and slip out underneath the door. I was soooooooooooooooo embarrassed.

The rest of the appointment went by in a blur. I think I gave some blood for some lab tests, as shortly after I got back to work, my doctor's office phoned to say, "Stop what you are doing, get in a cab and get yourself to emergency." Apparently I had appendicitis and my little pouch was ready to burst at any moment.

Had I known back then what I know now, I wouldn't have ended up in surgery, because my bowel would have been clean and functioning properly, and there would have been no chance of developing appendicitis.

There were lots of signs and signals my bowel needed attention, but it had never been dinner conversation in my household; and even if it was mentioned, no one in my circle of influence knew what proper bowel function was or how to correct it.

One of the signs and symptoms I ignored was my stinky feet, which were a direct result of my stinky colon. Still, I don't remember how irregularly I pooped. Obviously it wasn't enough, because the waste that should have been passing out was sitting in my colon, brewing up some very wretched smells, which were regularly escaping by way of fluffs, burps and, worst of all, via my feet.

Nothing helped my stinky feet, and boy did they stink. I used to wash them several times a day, put foot powder in my shoes, try different nylons and socks, but to no avail. My biggest fear in those days was I might be taken out on a date to a Japanese restaurant where I would have to take my shoes off outside one of those little booths. Then my date would be sniffing the air throughout the evening, eventually discovering the smell was coming from me.

If I had known back then what I know now, I never would have put myself through the grueling regime I followed in a vain effort to flatten out my tummy. Often I would look down at my abdomen and think I looked several months pregnant. Determined to do something about this problem, I went on yet another diet, which only served to ruin my metabolism. But, even at my ideal body weight I still had a very bulging abdomen. Being persistent I doubled up my efforts to flatten out my tummy. I began doing a minimum of 50 sit-ups a day and I still looked pregnant. I finally learned to live with it.

Not only was I ignorant about the functioning of my bowel, I was equally clueless about the female hormonal cycle. Oh, I understood about birth control and periods, but the phrase premenstrual syndrome (PMS) was foreign to me. I never clued in to why I would all of a sudden swell up like a water balloon and then 7-14 days later I would shrink again. These symptoms never had any rhyme or reason to me, and they just seemed to appear right out of the blue and then disappear just as mysteriously.

Sometimes my legs would bear the worst of my water retention and I could barely walk. No problem I thought, as I was so bitchy no one wanted to be around me anyways. So, I would just sit around, feeling irritable and depressed, eating everything sweet in sight. When those PMS cravings hit me, if there wasn't something sweet in the house, I would make a bowl of icing and eat it all. Makes my teeth hurt just thinking about it now.

By the time I had reached the age of 23, I was really a mess. I think I had every PMS symptom there was. Thankfully this was the age I started my nutrition career. I was very fortunate to be immediately introduced to the concept of "colon cleansing" (and I am not referring to colonic therapy, but to cleansing the colon with herbs and fiber).

I was shocked and dismayed at the amount of fecal material I eliminated. I won't go into those graphic details about the volume of waste leaving my body, but I like to joke around and say I even saw the pink Barbie shoe I swallowed when I was six.

Anyway, the colon cleanse was nothing short of miraculous. It got rid of my stinky feet (as well as the burps and fluffs), and it flattened my bulging abdomen; and best of all, my PMS vanished (until I started into my superwoman stress phase seven years later).

FAST AND SLOW

This is a fast track solution because if you can restore proper bowel function quickly, you can notice an immediate difference in your hormonal symptoms.

But, restoring proper bowel function can be a slow process, depending on how long you have had improper bowel function and how compliant you are with the suggestions I am going to make for you.

Plus there are two stages to restoring colon health.

Stage One: Improve day-to-day function to achieve elimination as close as possible to my description of proper bowel function. This should be a short process but some women have very stubborn bowels that resist even the best efforts to "reform."

Stage Two: Remove all of the old fecal material. You will need the right combination of herbs and supplemental fiber, along with very specific instructions on "how to cleanse" (no special diet, fasting or colonics required). If done properly, this stage will typically take at least six weeks to three months.

I am going to give you as much support as possible for stage one, but for stage two you will need either:

a) Assistance from your health care practitioner

b) A detailed manual on the cleansing process
   (refer to www.HormoneRollerCoaster.com)

HELP WITH STAGE ONE

Since starting the **Fast Track Foundation**, you may have noticed you are eliminating better already.

Here are the steps you have already taken towards improved bowel function.

1. Problem: Magnesium Deficiency

Calcium causes contraction and magnesium stimulates release so if you are high in calcium or low in magnesium, the result could be the contracted state of constipation.

Solution: You are supplementing appropriately with magnesium citrate.

2. Problem: Nutritional Deficiences

A deficiency of any nutrient can have a negative impact on the function of any of your glands and organs, including your bowel.

Solution: By supplementing with the Daily Essential Nutrients, you are nourishing your body in a way that is also supportive of proper bowel function.

Here are just a FEW of the nutrients supporting healthy bowel function.

- Alfalfa is the richest land source of trace minerals. This helps your body maintain a proper pH balance. It is also a good source of fiber.
- B1 - A deficiency of thiamine (B1) can cause constipation.
- Niacin (B3) is vital to the formation and maintenance of healthy digestive system tissues.
- Vitamin A helps repair the mucous membranes of your intestinal tract.
- Buffered vitamin C with bioflavanoids protects against bacterial infections.
- MSM (methyl-sulfonyl-methane) is particularly useful for people who have food allergies, inflammatory conditions, have lost the elasticity in their colon or have small portions of stretched intestines such as diverticulitis and hemorrhoids.

MSM is beneficial to these conditions because it helps your cells become more permeable, which allows toxins out of the cells and nutrients in. This allows for better healing and reduces food sensitivities. MSM can help restore flexibility and elasticity, which helps bring back some tone to your overstretched colon.

3. Problem: Candida Overgrowth

You should have about 4 to 8 lbs of friendly bacteria in your bowel which will do many things for you. This includes creating lubricated bulky stools which, in turn, will prevent constipation.

Solution: By treating yourself for a Candida overgrowth (if you had one) you will have rebalanced your intestinal bacteria, which will have gone a long way towards improving your day-to-day bowel function.

3. Problem: Stress

Stress, anxiety or any strong emotion will be interpreted by the body as an emergency situation. Energy will be diverted away from digestive functions. The result can be a slowing or stopping of all digestive activities including the motion of the colon.

Occasionally, the result may be quite the opposite, with a powerful and explosive wave-like action causing sudden diarrhea.

Solution: If you have identified stress is an underlying problem, you will have already taken the appropriate action as outlined in Chapter 10: **Fast Track Solution Five - Restore Adrenal Balance**.

NOW IT IS TIME TO ADDRESS YOUR LIFESTYLE

If you haven't already done so, please bookmark this spot and go now to the **Lifestyle Strategies For A Lifetime**, chapters 15 to 22. These chapters will give you additional assistance with phase one: improving day-to-day function to achieve elimination as close as possible to my description of proper bowel function.

CHAPTER 12

Fast Track Solution Seven: Reversing An Iodine Deficiency and Subclinical Hypothyroidism

The trace mineral iodine is important to women's hormones in three critical ways.

1. Iodine can reduce estrogen dominance by helping to protect women from a surge in the production of estrogen.

2. It desensitizes estrogen receptors in the breast tissue, which in turn can reduce the incidence of fibrocystic breast disease and breast cancer.

3. It aids in the development and functioning of the thyroid gland.

However, in the words of iodine specialist Dr. David Brownstein, "The role of iodine in the body goes far beyond its function of making thyroid hormones. Iodine is related to the ability to resist disease. Iodine is not only necessary for the production of thyroid hormone; it is also responsible for the production of all the other hormones in the body."

And Dr. George Flechas, who specializes in Iodine Therapy for thyroid and breast disorders, wrote, "Iodine is utilized by every hormone receptor in the body. The absence of iodine causes a hormonal dysfunction that can be seen with practically every hormone inside the body."

Given the importance of iodine, you will want to make sure you are not deficient.

How can you tell?

Most iodine deficiencies show up as subclinical hypothyroid symptoms.

My definition for the term subclinical hypothyroidism is: *when the body has symptoms of hypothyroidism but the blood tests do not confirm this condition.*

It is hard to estimate the true number of people who are suffering with subclinical hypothyroidism.

Dr. Thierry Hertoghe, President of the International Hormone Society (the third largest hormone society in the world with over 2,300 physicians as members) states, "many studies are now showing that people with levels of thyroid hormones (T4 and T3) in the lower fifth, quarter, third or half of the reference range and levels within the upper fifth, quarter, third or half of the TSH reference range have an increased risk of disease or even mortality."

Dr. Hertoghe's statement explains exactly what I am describing: the blood work falls within the normal range, YET, the risk of disease is higher because the person is actually hypothyroid. Until thyroid testing and parameters change, we will need to refer to this condition as subclinical hypothyroidism.

It is also Dr. Thierry Hertoghe's opinion that thyroid deficiency is prevalent in 20% to 50% (20 - 50 people in every 100) of a standard population.

DO YOU HAVE SUBCLINICAL HYPOTHYROID SYMPTOMS?

Following is a list of typical symptoms (a printable version is available at www.HormoneRollerCoaster.com).

Put an x beside every symptom you currently have.

____ Muscles stiff in morning; feel the need to limber up

____ Feel creaky after sitting still for periods of time

____ Heart sometimes seems to miss beats or turn "flip-flops"**

____ Coughing, hoarseness and/or muscle cramps that worsen at night

____ Dizzy or nauseated in the morning

____ Low energy, fatigue, lethargy, need lots of sleep (more than eight hours), trouble getting up and going in the morning

____ Motion sickness when traveling, dizzy when changing up and down positions**

____ Tendency to feel cold, particularly in hands and feet

____ Hair scanty, dry, brittle, lusterless

____ Dry skin**

____ Sleeplessness, restlessness

____ Usually less than one daily bowel movement**

____ Loss of libido**

____ Gain weight easily, fail to lose on diets**

____ Poor concentration or memory, mental sluggishness

____ Clogged sinuses

____ Low blood pressure/low pulse rate

____ Chronic low body temperature, especially at complete bed rest**

____ Recurrent infections

____ Menstrual problems including excessive bleeding, severe cramping, irregular periods, severe PMS, scanty flow; early or late onset of first period (before 12 or after 14 years old); premenopausal cessation of menstruation

___ Depression (including postpartum or after the start of menstruation or menopause)

___ Headaches (including migraines)

___ Family history of thyroid problems

___ Weight gain began when you got your period, had a miscarriage or an abortion, gave birth, began menopause, or worsened after low-calorie dieting

___ Chubby or overweight since childhood

___ Hoarseness, gravelly voice**

___ Swollen eyelids and face, general water retention

___ Thinning or loss of outside eyebrow hair**

___ High cholesterol

___ Lump in throat, trouble swallowing pills**

___ Slow body movement or speech**

___ Muscle and joint pain, or carpal tunnel syndrome**

___ Dry/gritty eyes

If you have eight x's or more, especially if you have at least two or three of the symptoms marked with a double asterisk (**), you should consider following the upcoming protocol for thyroid support.

Also, if you have fibrocystic breast disease or ovarian cysts, or a uterine fibroid, I would highly recommend adding some form of supplemental iodine to your daily regime.

How Much Iodine Should You Add?

My clinical experience has been limited to the dosages available to me in Canada.

The Norwegian kelp product I have been suggesting to clients for years only contains 455 mcg of iodine per capsule and I routinely suggest 5 capsules twice a day.

I like kelp because it provides a natural source of iodine and is a good promoter of glandular health. Kelp contains nearly 30 minerals, so it is also helpful for adding vital trace minerals.

My recommendation will give you 4.5 mg of iodine daily. Is that enough? The answer depends on whom you ask. It could be lots or could be considered just a mere drop in the bucket.

Anyone in the traditional medical field will stick to the Recommended Daily Allowance (RDA) for iodine which is 150 micrograms daily for everybody over the age of 14. With everything we know today about iodine, this amount seems absurdly low.

In his book, *Iodine, Bringing Back the Universal Medicine*, Dr. Mark Sircus explains, "One of the last essential elements included in the RDA system was iodine, established in 1980 and confirmed in 1989. The RDA for iodine was based on the amount of iodine/iodide needed to prevent goiter, extreme stupidity and hypothyroidism. The optimal requirement of the whole human body for iodine has never been studied. Therefore, the optimal amount of this element for physical and mental wellbeing is unknown. Based on demographic studies, the mainland Japanese consumed an average of 13.8 mg daily and they are one of the healthiest people on planet earth."

The RDA has never changed. Why would it? There is no profit in finding ways to keep people healthy with food and nutritional supplements as opposed to the billions of dollars to be made by selling people drugs to treat their illnesses.

So, we must depend on the pioneers in nutritional research to guide us.

Drs. Abraham, Flechas and Brownstein tested more than 4,000 patients taking iodine in daily doses ranging from 12.5 to 50 mg, and in those with diabetes, up to 100 mg a day. These investigators found that *iodine does indeed reverse fibrocystic disease; their diabetic patients require less insulin; hypothyroid patients, less thyroid medication; symptoms of fibromyalgia resolve, and patients with migraine headaches stop having them.* Dr. Mark Sircus adds, "We can expect even better results when iodine is combined with magnesium."

Dr. David Derry wrote, *"Lugol's solution is an iodine-in-water solution used by the medical profession for 200 years. One drop (6.5 mg of iodine per drop) of Lugol's daily in water, orange juice or milk will gradually eliminate the first phase of the cancer development namely fibrocystic disease of the breast so no new cancers can start. It also will kill abnormal cells floating around in the body at remote sites from the original cancer. Of course this approach appears to work for prostate cancer as prostate cancer is similar to breast cancer in many respects. Indeed, it likely will help with most cancers. Also higher doses of iodine are required for inflammatory breast cancer. As well we know that large doses of intravenous iodine are harmless which makes one wonder what effect this would have on cancer growth."*

Dr. H. Duffy Sr. wrote, *"I was shrinking tumors in the early seventies by using thousands of times the RDA of Iodine. Iodine along with the proper essential fat and additional vitamins will fix just about any thyroid problem."*

Dr. David Miller wrote, *"Iodine is needed in microgram amounts for the thyroid, mg amounts for breast and other tissues, and can be used therapeutically in gram amounts."*

Dr. David Brownstein, in his book, *Iodine: Why You Need It; Why You Can't Live Without It,* says, *"Of all the elements known so far to be essential for human health, iodine is the most misunderstood and the most feared. Yet, iodine is the safest of all the essential trace elements, being the only one that can be administered safely for long periods of time to large numbers of patients in daily amounts as high as 100,000 times the RDA. However, this safety record only applies to inorganic, non-radioactive forms of iodine. Some organic iodine containing drugs are extremely toxic and prescribed by physicians. The severe side effects of these drugs are blamed on inorganic iodine although studies have clearly demonstrated that it is the whole molecule that is toxic, not the iodine released from it."*

So it would seem there is a wide range of possibilities, and it will depend on what you are hoping to accomplish and what you feel comfortable taking.

Conclusion On Iodine Deficiency

I have witnessed no ill effects, only positive benefits, with clients taking 6 to 10 capsules (in divided doses) of Norwegian Kelp (each capsule containing 455 mcg of iodine) daily.

People with Hashimoto's Thyroiditis should not introduce kelp into their regime without the guidance of a qualified health care practitioner.

If your doctor has tested you for low thyroid and the results have come back negative, then you do not have Hashimoto's Thyroiditis.

TWO CAUTIONS:

1. Allergic Reaction: It isn't common but is possible to have an allergic reaction to iodine, so you should start with a small test amount before increasing your dosage.

If you take kelp (or any other iodine supplement) and experience an allergic reaction such as itching, skin rash, hives, watery or itchy eyes, runny nose, or shortness of breath, stop taking the product. If you are unsure if your symptoms are related to the kelp, wait until all the symptoms have cleared and then you can try it again.

2. Hashimoto's Thyroiditis: Is an autoimmune inflammatory process, which means the body creates antibodies which attack the thyroid gland, resulting in a deficiency of thyroid hormone.

The symptoms of Hashimoto's Thyroiditis are similar to those of hypothyroidism in general, which are often subtle. They are not specific (which means they can mimic the symptoms of many other conditions) and are often attributed to aging. The symptoms generally become more obvious as the condition worsens and the majority of these complaints are related to a slowing of metabolic process in the body.

Common symptoms are:

- Fatigue
- Depression
- Modest weight gain
- Cold intolerance, feeling cold
- Excessive sleepiness
- Dry, coarse hair or thinning hair
- Constipation
- Dry skin
- Muscle cramps
- Increased cholesterol levels
- Decreased concentration
- Vague aches and pains
- Swelling of the legs
- Pale, puffy face
- Heavy menstrual flow or irregular periods
- A slowed heart rate
- Problems getting pregnant

Other symptoms and signs include:

- Swelling of the thyroid gland (due to the inflammation), leading to a feeling of tightness or fullness in the throat
- A lump in the front of the neck, (the enlarged thyroid gland) called a goiter
- Difficulty swallowing solids and/or liquids, due to the enlargement of the thyroid gland

If you have symptoms of Hashimoto's Thyroiditis, go to your doctor and ask for a TSH (thyroid stimulating hormone) and an antibody test.

People with Hashimoto's Thyroiditis will have:

1. An above-normal level of TSH, which is a sign of an under-active thyroid along with:

2. The specific antibodies that people with other causes of an underactive thyroid do not have.

The strategies for supporting subclinical low thyroid are safe, but if you are diagnosed with Hashimoto's Thyroiditis, do not start on any iodine until you have consulted with your health care practitioner.

KEY STEPS TO OVERCOMING SUBCLINICAL HYPOTHYROIDISM

Adding an iodine supplement to your regime is just one step in overcoming subclinical hypothyroidism.

The great news is if you have been using this book as suggested and taking action where appropriate for you, then you won't have a lot of work left to do.

If not, then you will see there is a substantial amount of work to be done and you will find it far less overwhelming to go back to chapter 1 and start at the beginning, taking one step at a time.

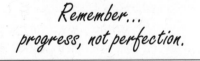

Remember...
progress, not perfection.

OTHER REQUIRED NUTRIENTS FOR OPTIMAL THYROID FUNCTION

When you view the following list, I hope you will be excited to see you have been getting all of these nutrients since the day you began taking the **Fast Track Foundation**.

1. Selenium and Zinc

Selenium is crucial in both the production of T-4 thyroid hormone (thyroxine) in the thyroid gland, as well as in the conversion of T-4 to T-3 thyroid hormone, the active form (thyronine). Zinc is needed both before and after these production and conversion processes. Zinc is necessary for the TRH (thyrotropin-releasing hormone) produced by the hypothalamus to stimulate the pituitary gland, which signals the thyroid gland to produce thyroid hormone.

Both selenium and zinc are included in the Daily Essential Nutrients. However, there are times when you may need to take an extra selenium and/or zinc supplement. If you follow all of the protocols in this book and still show multiple subclinical hypothyroid symptoms, then I would definitely seek the assistance of a qualified health care practitioner to see if extra zinc and/or selenium are what you require.

2. Vitamin D

Vitamin D is necessary for thyroid hormone production in the pituitary gland. You need at least 800 international units (IU) of vitamin D daily to support thyroid function.

There is 500 IU of vitamin D3 suggested in the Daily Essentials Nutrients. Usually you can get the balance from adequate sun exposure but sometimes additional vitamin D3 supplementation is necessary.

Vitamin D3 is produced in the body when ultraviolet rays from sunlight strike the skin. At least 75% of the body's supply comes from conversion in the skin. You can make 10,000 to 12,000 IU of vitamin D in just half an hour. So whenever possible, get daily direct sunshine for at least five minutes, and make sure you don't completely cover your body whenever you're outside.

Keep in mind that wearing sunscreen pretty much voids the ability of your skin to produce vitamin D from sunlight – meaning, the more you cover up and/or use sunscreen, the more you need to supplement.

3. Vitamin E

Besides the key benefits of vitamin E listed in Chapter 6: **Daily Essential Nutrients**, 400-800 IU daily is also required for optimizing your thyroid function.

4. Magnesium

You can't make ANY hormones without enough magnesium. You not only get some in your Daily Essential Nutrients, but you are taking an additional magnesium supplement (if appropriate for you).

5. Other Nutrients

You need a host of other nutrients as well, but all of these (such as vitamin A, omega 3, and antioxidants) are provided for you in the Daily Essential Nutrients.

L-Tyrosine is NOT included.

L-Tyrosine is an amino acid your thyroid uses to make its vital metabolic regulators, T3 and T4. These hormones stimulate every cell in your body, including your brain cells.

If you follow all the protocols in this book and still show multiple sub-clinical hypothyroid symptoms, then I would definitely seek the assistance of a qualified health care practitioner to see if extra L-Tyrosine is what you require.

In the interim, it would be very helpful to make sure you are eating foods rich in L-Tyrosine.

Meats: lamb, veal, beef, chicken, turkey, as well as wild game such as quail, duck and ostrich. Most fish have high levels of L-Tyrosine, including orange roughy, tuna, shrimp and cod.

Fruits and Vegetables: Seaweed has one of the highest levels of L-Tyrosine. Green foods such as spinach, mustard greens and pumpkin seeds also have healthy amounts of L-Tyrosine. Eating avocados is a great way to get a boost of L-Tyrosine.

Nuts, Seeds, Beans and Grains: Nuts such as almonds, as well as sesame seeds and pumpkin seeds, and whole grains such as wheat and oats contain L-Tyrosine. Other sources include kidney and lima beans.

OTHER FACTORS THAT INFLUENCE THYROID FUNCTION

1. Estrogen Dominance

If you are estrogen dominant, then you won't utilize your thyroid hormones properly.

Everything I have been suggesting so far is focused on lowering excess estrogen and balancing it with progesterone.

2. Adrenal Fatigue

Your adrenal glands and your thyroid are intimately linked. This means subclinical hypothyroidism is almost always preceded by some level of adrenal fatigue.

You can't restore thyroid function without rejuvenating your adrenal glands.

If you skipped through Chapter 10: **Fast Track Solution Five - Restore Adrenal Balance**, it is time to go back and review it in depth.

3. Liver Dysfunction

A healthy liver will convert the thyroid hormone thyroxin (T4) into its more active form, thyronine (T3). Inadequate conversion of T4 to T3 by the liver may lead to hypothyroidism, chronic fatigue, weight gain, poor memory, and a host of other problems.

We will cover this topic in the next chapter. Soon you will see you have taken many steps already to support your liver function.

LIFESTYLE STRATEGIES

If you haven't yet read **Lifestyle Strategies For A Lifetime**, chapters 15 to 22, please put a bookmark in this spot and go there now. Pay particular attention to these two topics as they relate very specifically to thyroid health.

1. Soy Foods: Review Chapter 18: Lifestyle Strategy Four

Unfermented soy products interfere with thyroid function. The only safe soy food to include in your diet is organic and fermented in the forms of tempeh, miso, natto, as well as some fermented soy sauces.

Do not eat tofu, soy cheese, soy milk, soy dogs, soy protein, etc, as they are not fermented.

2. Fluoride: Review Chapter 22: Lifestyle Strategy Eight

Excerpt from **The Effects Of Fluoride On The Thyroid Gland**
By Dr Barry Durrant-Peatfield MBBS LRCP MRCS
Medical Advisor to Thyroid UK

"It has been known since the latter part of the 19th century that certain communities, notably in Argentina, India and Turkey were chronically ill, with premature ageing, arthritis, mental retardation, and infertility; and high levels of natural fluorides in the water were responsible. Not only was it clear that the fluoride was having a general effect on the health of the community, but in the early 1920s Goldemberg, working in Argentina showed that fluoride was displacing iodine; thus compounding the damage and rendering the community also hypothyroid from iodine deficiency."

The Method To My 'Madness'

In this chapter, I have illustrated how I have been expertly guiding you step by step through the health balancing actions you need to take to resolve ALL of your hormone issues, including subclinical hypothyroidism.

What My Clients Have to Say About Kelp

THANKS Brenda for suggesting Kelp. I had hoped it would help me lose weight and so far I haven't lost but then again, I haven't put on any more either (I have been on a steady increase lately due to stress). But the great new is I usually have VERY heavy menstrual cycles with lots of clotting...for the first time in 2 years, it didn't happen. I stopped the progesterone cream, started the kelp. I usually go through 2 boxes super plus tampons (in addition to pads), and not this time. I know the kelp made the difference. Thanks again.

–Heidi H, Hazard, Kentucky, US

My periods are back like clockwork since taking 10 kelp a day! Thank you once again!

–Caroline W, Qualicum Beach, BC

CHAPTER 13

Fast Track Solution Eight:
Support Optimal Liver Function

In this chapter, I am going to explain the relationship between your liver and your hormones.

It Is Not What You Think

Many women never consider their liver could be contributing to their health and hormonal issues. They also believe if they do have a liver issue, their doctor will inform them.

The first misconception usually stems from the myth, "if you aren't a heavy drinker (alcohol), you have no need for concern."

Most women assume alcohol is the leading cause of stress to their livers; and although it is a stress, it isn't the biggest one. Someone who has never touched a drop of alcohol can be just as much at risk of liver dysfunction as someone who drinks moderately. Toxins and nutritional deficiencies are the real troublemakers.

The second misconception stems from the fact there are blood tests any doctor can administer for liver function. But these tests will only tell you if your liver is suffering from an infectious disease or severe drug and alcohol related liver damage. Unfortunately, a large amount of liver tissue must be damaged or destroyed before the customary tests of liver function reveal abnormality. Unless you have outright liver disease, these tests aren't the best indicators of liver function.

So once again, I am referring to a subclinical state in which no outright disease exists, yet the liver is not functioning optimally. I refer to this as "liver dysfunction" or "subclinical liver dysfunction."

In the case of liver dysfunction, you can be suffering with a whole host of symptoms which relate to the over 500 functions your liver performs for you.

I am only listing a *few* I feel have the *greatest* relevance to your hormonal concerns.

1. Hormone Balance

The liver plays a <u>huge</u> role in keeping your hormones balanced by breaking down what's left of the hormones after they have served their messenger function to their target cells.

a. Reducing Estrogen Dominance

This means your liver will "dispose" of estrogen after it has been used. If the liver does not metabolize estrogen properly, estrogen dominance can result in the very list of symptoms you are trying to eliminate.

b. Water Retention

Aldosterone is a hormone released by the adrenal glands. It increases the reabsorption of sodium and water and the release of potassium in the kidneys. If the liver does not break down aldosterone efficiently, water retention can be the result.

c. Mood Control

Stress (real or perceived) causes adrenaline to pump through your veins. Physical exertion is one way to use up adrenaline, but as mentioned above, your liver can also dispose of these hormones once they have served their messenger purpose. Failure to dispose of adrenaline after it has outlived its usefulness may lead to chronic irritability and temper explosions.

> *The liver is known metaphysically*
> *as the "seat of anger"*

2. Menopausal Support (for the perimenopausal woman)

Liver dysfunction can cause menopausal symptoms to be more severe.

There are three types of estrogen: estriol, estrone and estradiol. Estriol primarily affects a woman's hair, nails, skin, and her vaginal lining. When a woman goes through menopause, the estrogen production from the ovaries is dramatically reduced, and it is primarily up to the adrenal glands to produce the back-up supply. However, a healthy liver can also produce small amounts of estriol which goes a long way in helping eliminate any menopausal symptoms.

3. Fat Control

Your liver is largely responsible for whether you store fat or burn fat, including the fat on your body (predominately your belly).

4. Thyroid Function

A healthy liver will convert the thyroid hormone thyroxin (T4) into its more active form (T3). Inadequate conversion of T4 to T3 by the liver may lead to hypothyroidism, chronic fatigue, weight gain, poor memory, and a host of other problems.

Problem: Toxins

Our toxic lifestyles have the biggest impact on our livers. Toxic substances are everywhere. You are bombarded with toxins in the air you breathe, the food you eat, in the products you apply to your skin, the water you drink and every drug you take. Even the bad bacteria in your intestines produce toxic substances, all of which must be removed from your blood and neutralized by your liver.

Just as the filter in your car gets clogged from use, so does your liver. If you never changed the filter in your car, would you expect it to run properly? What about your water purifier? If you never changed it, how pure would your water be? How would it taste? Would it contain harmful toxins and bacteria?

I am not suggesting you exchange your liver for a new one, like you change the filters in your car, furnace and water purifiers. I am just using these analogies to help you see how your liver can be swamped with work. An overload of toxins interferes with its function.

Solution: Great news! You have already been working on them.

1. You are drinking more water, which helps flush toxins from your body. Review Chapter 15: **Lifestyle Strategy One**.

2. You have reduced your exposure to toxic xenoestrogens. Review Chapter 19: **Lifestyle Strategy Five**.

3. You have reduced your exposure to toxic fluoride. Review Chapter 22: **Lifestyle Strategy Eight**.

4. Candida yeast ferments sugars into acetaldehyde, which is the same carcinogen that causes alcohol hangovers. Candida also increases levels of ammonia, which is another liver toxin.

   Candida overgrowth is toxic but this should not be a problem for you now. If you identified a Candida overgrowth, you will have already completed the treatment to eradicate the excess. Review Chapter 9: **Fast Track Solution Four - Eliminate a Candida Overgrowth**.

5. Improper bowel function can create some of the most toxic chemicals known to mankind. Since your intestines are designed to absorb nutrients, along with those nutrients you also absorb the residual toxins from your colon into your bloodstream, which must then be filtered through your liver.

   Again this is an area you have already been paying huge attention to. Review Chapter 11: **Fast Track Solution Six - Ensure Proper Bowel Function**.

Problem: Lack of Nutrients

The liver is an amazing organ and can usually regenerate if the diet is adequate in supplying all essential nutrients. Unfortunately, as discussed in Chapter Three: **Do We Really Need Vitamins**, the average modern-day diet does not provide the nutrients your liver needs to maintain optimal function.

Solution: More great news! The **Daily Essential Nutrients**, which you have already been taking, provide those essential nutrients your liver requires for good health. They include:

1. **B complex Vitamins**: essential for healthy metabolic functioning. Working individually and synergistically, they facilitate energy release and the manufacture of new cells.

   Choline, in particular, helps reduce the amount of fat deposited in the liver.

2. **Antioxidants**: afford protection to the liver from the damaging effects of free radicals produced from environmental toxins. The best antioxidants for the liver are:

   Vitamin C (as calcium ascorbate): protects the liver. Even doses as low as 500 milligrams daily help prevent fatty buildup and cirrhosis (much more serious diseases than "liver dysfunction").

   Vitamin E and the trace minerals selenium and zinc.

3. **MSM** (methyl-sulfonyl-methane): the richest source of organic sulfur available. Sulfur is integral in the formation of bile acids by the liver. It must be present in the body for it to make its own antioxidant, Glutathione, which is extremely important for detoxifying the liver.

4. **Omega 3**: helps the liver to reduce the inflammation of its cells, which aids in its natural healing process.

5. **Green Tea**: protects the liver from the negative effects of toxic substances such as alcohol. Green tea's catechins are helpful in reducing liver inflammation. Green tea helps to cleanse the

liver. Although your liver doesn't actually need this, you can see why it is very beneficial.

Assistance from B6 and/or I-3-C

You have already been assisting your liver to clear excess estrogen by taking additional B6 and/or I-3-C since you started the **Fast Track Foundation**.

No One Is Immune

No matter how healthy you are, your liver works hard for you and it could use all the TLC it can get.

Since you can't take your filter (liver) out of your body to clean it, I highly recommend giving it some extra support.

This can be accomplished safely and easily with the herb Milk Thistle. The ingredient list on the Milk Thistle you choose should read between 150 and 200 mg of Milk Thistle Seed Extract with a standardized minimum of 75% silymarin.

Silymarin not only prevents the depletion of glutathione, but has also been shown to increase the level of glutathione in the liver.

Glutathione in the liver is critically linked to the liver's ability to detoxify. The higher the glutathione content, the greater the liver's capacity to detoxify harmful chemicals/toxins.

Typically, the more chemicals/toxins you are exposed to, the more the concentration of glutathione in the liver is reduced. This reduction in glutathione makes the liver cells susceptible to damage and disease.

Milk Thistle is one of the most effective nutrients for regenerating liver function, because it increases production of new liver cells to replace the old damaged ones. It is extremely safe to use.

Note: *If you are allergic to ragweed, chrysanthemums, marigolds, chamomile, yarrow, or daisies, you could be allergic to Milk Thistle.*

How to Take Milk Thistle

There are no hard and fast rules about how much or how long a person should support and cleanse her liver. Rather than stating maximums, I am giving you minimums. We know that Milk Thistle is safe to use for longer periods of time because of its track record. Milk Thistle extracts have been used as traditional herbal remedies for almost 2,000 years. The only people who should not use it are those who have an allergy to the plant itself or other plants in the aster family.

You can take 1 capsule daily for a little extra liver "boost," or you can give your liver major support starting with 1 capsule a day, and slowly over a period of a couple of weeks, increase your dosage by increments of 1 capsule until you are taking 2 capsules twice a day.

The rate at which you increase your dosage of Milk Thistle depends on whether or not you are experiencing any cleansing reactions. You might feel fatigued or experience flu-like symptoms. If these occur, it is a sign of cleansing (which is what you want to happen). Don't be discouraged, and don't increase your dosage until those symptoms pass. Allow at least four to five days at each new dosage before deciding on whether or not to increase.

If you are going with a lower dose, then you will want to stay with Milk Thistle for at least 90 days. If you choose the major support, stay with it for a minimum of 30 days.

Considering the significant role your liver plays in keeping you healthy and balancing your hormones, I truly feel you should consider a Milk Thistle "boost" or major support at least once a year. You could also do the initial major support for longer than my 30-day minimum recommendation.

A Client Comment About Liver Support

I was taking your product with Milk Thistle for my liver awhile back and it really seemed to help with my sore breasts. Since I haven't been taking it, they have been getting increasingly sorer every month. I obviously did not stay on it long enough and will go back on it to correct the problem.

–Vicki R, Red Deer, Alta

CHAPTER 14

Fast Track Solution Nine:
The Appropriate Use of Natural
Bio-Identical Progesterone Cream

Please read this chapter carefully as there is a lot of information you need to know in order to utilize progesterone cream safely and effectively.

First, what is natural progesterone cream?

Natural progesterone cream is also referred to as bio-identical progesterone because it is the identical hormone women produce. I use the entire phrase "natural bio-identical progesterone cream" because some bio-identical progesterone is not in a non-toxic carrier so you can't really call it "natural."

Some women think they are getting bio-identical progesterone when they take birth control pills or Provera (synthetic form of progesterone), but they aren't. Birth control pills and Provera contain progestin, which is synthetic, and not at all the same as bio-identical progesterone.

Progestin has a long list of negative side effects as bad as, if not worse than, those produced by estrogen dominance. For a complete list of progestin side effects, please go to www.HormoneRollerCoaster.com

Another common misunderstanding is that wild yam herb will do the same thing for you as bio-identical progesterone cream. This is not true.

Wild yam herb contains a substance called diosgenin, which can only be made into bio-identical progesterone through a chemical process in a laboratory. Your body cannot do this.

Earlier in this book, I suggested wild yam as one of the herbs you could take to help rejuvenate your adrenal glands. I did not suggest it hoping your body would be able to convert the diosgenin into bio-identical progesterone. Only chemists can make this conversion – your body can't.

Remember that wild yam herb is for supporting your adrenal glands and is not a source of bio-identical progesterone. Because the purpose of using natural bio-identical progesterone cream is different than the purpose of taking the wild yam herb, you can safely use them both at the same time.

Many women purchase wild yam cream thinking they are getting bio-identical progesterone cream, but they aren't. Even though the wild yam herb found in the wild yam cream is delivered to your bloodstream via your skin, your body still can't convert the diosgenin into bio-identical progesterone. If you have found relief by using wild yam cream, it is because of the support the wild yam herb gives to your adrenal glands and not because the wild yam cream has provided you with bio-identical progesterone.

Who Should Use Progesterone Cream?

I don't recommend progesterone cream for everyone, so the following information will help sort out who should use bio-identical prog-esterone cream and who shouldn't.

You **CANNOT** use bio-identical progesterone cream if you are cur-rently using any form of progestin such as birth control pills or prog-estin in hormone replacement therapy such as Provera.

You **CANNOT** use bio-identical progesterone cream if you have an IUD such as Mirena, as it releases progestin into your body. (In my opinion no woman should be using this type of IUD PERIOD!)

You SHOULD NOT use bio-identical progesterone cream if you are using Prometrium, which is the pharmaceutical version of natural progesterone in pill form. I personally prefer the natural progesterone cream over Prometrium.

I also do not advocate the use of bio-identical progesterone cream for women under the age of 32, unless recommended by a qualified health care practitioner.

For everyone else, my rule of thumb is, if you have mild to moderate symptoms of PMS, try balancing your hormones without using progesterone cream. If you have severe PMS or moderate to severe perimenopause with any of the following symptoms, I suggest you begin using natural bio-identical progesterone cream as soon as possible along with the rest of the strategies from this book.

- severe hot flashes/night sweats
- endometriosis
- fibroids
- infertility
- prone to miscarriages
- hormonally induced migraines
- excessive heavy periods and/or clotting
- extreme menstrual cramping

Progesterone Cream Is Not A Band-Aid Solution

I am in favor of natural bio-identical progesterone cream as an addition to your hormone balancing regime when appropriate BUT I am not in favor of using it instead of the strategies I indicate to nourish and rebalance your body.

If you use bio-identical progesterone cream without following any of the other recommendations in this book, then I have failed to impress upon you the true origin of disease.

If you choose only bio-identical progesterone (no fast track solutions and lifestyle changes), you will likely get at least some benefit. I am not denying that. My point is this: relying solely on bio-identical progesterone (or any other bio-identical hormone) means you are ignoring your body's attempts to get your attention.

Every one of your symptoms is a cry for help from your body. Ignore the cries and your body will find other ways of getting your attention.

For example: you are bleeding so heavily you decide a hysterectomy is your only recourse; instead, you use a liberal amount of bio-identical progesterone cream (but no other **Fast Track Solutions** or **Lifestyle Strategies for a Lifetime**) and your bleeding stops. You may wonder what is wrong with this scenario as you achieved the desired result, right?

Yes, you did, sort of. Consider this. We know the bleeding was caused by estrogen dominance, and let's say in this scenario the estrogen dominance was caused by improper bowel function. Because you chose to ignore the underlying root cause of the bleeding (improper bowel function leading to estrogen dominance) by not following the **Fast Track Solutions** and **Lifestyle Changes for a Lifetime**, your body will now have to find another way to get you to pay attention to your bowel.

This new cry for help could be psoriasis, severe abdominal bloating, irritable bowel syndrome or in the worst case scenario, colon cancer.

Another example would look like this. What if the estrogen dominance was because you were tiring out your adrenal glands trying to win an award for Superwoman of the Year?

In this scenario, you decided to bypass the adrenal rejuvenation section in favor of solely using natural bio-identical progesterone cream. Your body may start to cry out with symptoms such as hay fever, blood sugar swings, and in the worst case scenario, Chronic Fatigue Syndrome.

So yes, feel free to use bio-identical progesterone, but use it wisely. Please make sure it is only one part of your complete **Fast Track Solution** Program.

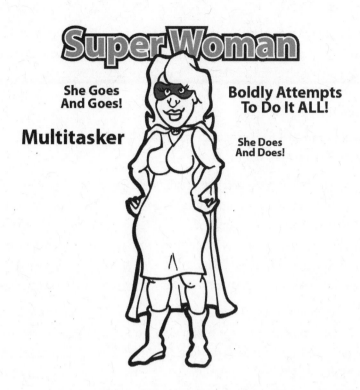

Super Woman

She Goes
And Goes!

Boldly Attempts
To Do It ALL!

Multitasker

She Does
And Does!

How to Use Natural Bio-identical Progesterone Cream

Where do you apply it?

Because bio-identical progesterone cream is absorbed into the skin and taken up by the fatty layer beneath, it is best absorbed where the skin is relatively thin and well supplied with capillary blood flow. Areas such as your face, neck, upper chest, breasts, inner arms, inside thighs, backs of the knees and palms of the hands are best suited for this. It is then transferred into the bloodstream where it circulates to progesterone receptor sites throughout your body.

Always rotate the application sites. In other words, don't apply the bio-identical progesterone cream to the same spot every day. For example, one day apply to your neck, the next day to the backs of your knees, the next day to the inside of your arms, then to your breasts and then the next day back to your neck again.

The amount you use and when you use it varies from woman to woman. I can't cover every possible circumstance but the following information should provide a solid guideline for the majority of women.

When do you use it?

A quality bio-identical progesterone cream will contain 400 to 600 mg. of progesterone per ounce.

The bio-identical progesterone cream I am familiar with contains 20 mg of pharmaceutical grade natural bio-identical progesterone in each ¼ teaspoon. Use anywhere from ⅛ to ½ teaspoon one to two times per day. The more severe the symptoms, the more bio-identical progesterone cream will likely be required. 20 mg of progesterone daily is the normal daily amount your ovaries would produce after ovulation.

To begin, count the first day of your period as day one. From day one to the day you ovulate (approximately mid-cycle) you are primarily producing estrogen; therefore, you should NOT be using progesterone cream during this time. Ovulation triggers the release of your own progesterone. Since you are trying to mimic the hormones of your cycle, you should be using the bio-identical progesterone cream from ovulation to the first day of your next period.

No matter how long your cycle is, you typically ovulate 14 days before your period. So, if day 1 is the first day of your period and you are going to get another period in 30 days, you would start the cream on day 17 or 18. If you are going to get a period in 24 days, you would start the cream on day 11 or 12. It is important to start using it AFTER you have ovulated. If you use it before you ovulate, then your own body may not produce its own progesterone.

Conversely, perimenopausal women experiencing severe bleeding along with short cycles (many women start getting periods every 24 days) are likely not ovulating every month, so my suggestion for these women is to start using the cream on day 10.

If you have very short cycles, you can expect the bio-identical progesterone cream to lengthen them over time, in which case you will need to adjust your application start date accordingly.

If you are trying to get pregnant and happen to conceive while using the bio-identical progesterone cream, continue to use the progesterone cream every day until the end of your third month, then very gradually wean off. Start by reducing the dosage by half, maintaining the dosage for one week and then repeat. If you were only using ½ teaspooon a day, then you would go to ¼ teaspoon a day for one week and then you can stop. When you are pregnant, your progesterone levels continue to rise. By the second trimester your body should be producing 400 mg of progesterone per day.

Dr. John Lee author of *What your Doctor May Not Tell You About Menopause* and *What Your Doctor May Not Tell You About Perimenopause* suggests women with endometriosis should use ¼ teaspoon of progesterone cream twice a day from day 6 to 14 and then ½ teaspoon twice a day from day 15 until just before your period is expected. Follow this program for six months, then discontinue using the cream from day 6 to day 14.

He also suggests if you have severe perimenopausal symptoms, e.g. if you are experiencing excessive bleeding, you can use ¼ teaspoon two times per day from day 8 to 21 and then ½ teaspoon two times per day from day 22 to the first day of your period. But if you are bleeding heavily AND getting your period every 24 days, start using ½ teaspoon twice a day from day 15 to the first day of your period.

If your specific needs do not fall into the outline I have provided, then please seek out the assistance of a health care practitioner who specializes in women's hormones.

Should you continue using progesterone cream indefinitely?

There are no "golden rules" as each woman is different. Women should use the progesterone cream (if appropriate) and follow the other **Fast**

Track Solutions and **Lifestyle Strategies for a Lifetime**. Once they feel like their hormones are in balance, they can cut their dosage in half and see how they feel during the next two cycles. If symptoms re-appear, they should go back to their previous dosage. If there is no reoccurrence of symptoms, they can stop using the cream altogether.

Generally, women who have not reached the perimenopausal phase (still ovulating and producing progesterone) are going to need the progesterone cream for less time than the perimenopausal women (not ovulating regularly and therefore not producing adequate amounts of progesterone).

Are there any side effects?

There are no known side effects of natural bio-identical progesterone when it is taken in small doses of 20 to 40 milligrams per day. Some women report a worsening of estrogen dominance symptoms the first week or two after starting progesterone. This is because the progesterone "wakes up" your estrogen sites, ultimately making better use of your circulating estrogen.

A temporary worsening of your symptoms is a clear indicator you are estrogen dominant and more progesterone, not less, is needed to offset the effects. Having given this warning, I want to ensure you that the majority of women feel immediately better when they start using progesterone cream, and only a small percentage of women experience a temporary worsening of symptoms, which pass in one to two weeks.

If you apply progesterone cream out of sync with your cycle, it may change the timing of your period, delay ovulation or cause some spotting mid-cycle. You cannot use progesterone cream to regulate your cycle as a form of birth control.

Where can you buy it?

Naturopaths and physicians in Canada can write prescriptions for natural bio-identical progesterone cream, and most compounding pharmacies can fill them.

In the United States, you can buy it directly from a health food store. Canadians are legally allowed to purchase it from the United States and import it for personal use.

If you can buy it off the shelf in Canada, it is not real bio-identical progesterone cream.

What My Clients Have To Say About Natural Bio-Identical Progesterone Cream

When I became perimenopausal about one year ago, I thought I was going to breeze through it with no problems at all, only periods every 4 months - I could live with that. Just before I went to Brenda's "For Women Only" full day workshop, I had a period that lasted full force for one month, and I thought I was going to bleed to death. When Brenda spoke about the Natural Progesterone Cream I knew it was for me - within 5 days of using the cream I had stopped bleeding. After combining this program with bowel cleansing, Essential Daily Nutrients and adrenal support, I no longer suffer from PMS, cramps or hormonal headaches. Thank you Brenda, for showing me the way to optimal health.

—Wendy S, Victoria, BC

I went to one of your hormone seminars and I just wanted to let you know that adding the progesterone cream to my regime worked like a miracle for my migraines. I have had cyclical migraines with my period every month from the age of 18-38. Then I went to my doctor and demanded a prescription for progesterone cream and it worked within 2 months - no migraines. Once again, thank you for helping me.

—Rosemary Q, Victoria, BC

LEANNE'S STORY

One of my Inner Circle members in the throes of perimenopause wrote:

I have been experiencing major issues with flow and clots. I feel like I am bleeding to death. Is there anything you can suggest? I am not sure why I didn't ask sooner - who knows. If I am honest, it is because I was waiting for it to just go away, but it is getting worse and not better. I swear that when there is something wrong with us, our brains fall out.

Because I had Leanne's file on hand, I was able to outline a plan of action which she started immediately. This is the email I sent to her:

Of course you are getting heavy periods and clots right now. It is really common for perimenopausal women to get heavy periods and clots. One of the functions of estrogen is to build the lining of your uterus known as your endometrium, but too much estrogen will create too much lining leading to problems such as endometriosis, heavy periods, clots and uterine fibroids.

Most perimenopausal women become EXCESSIVELY estrogen dominant before they stop their periods altogether. EXCESSIVE estrogen can mean EXCESSIVE periods and clots.

You are already taking the Daily Essential Nutrients so I am going to add the following.

Bio-identical progesterone will immediately balance out the estrogen dominance. I-3-C will work over the next few months, but will not give you the immediate results that you need.

I am suggesting kelp because you are iodine deficient, which results in you OVER-producing estrogen in perimenopause and under-producing estrogen in menopause.

Adrenal support for the stress this bleeding has caused you.

Magnesium for the hormone production and cramping.

Your program will look like this.

AM**bio-identical progesterone as outlined in the attachment.

After Breakfast:
  Daily Essentials
  1 B5
  5 kelp
  I-3-C

After lunch or dinner:
  Daily Essentials
  1 B5
  5 kelp
  I-3-C

Before bed:
  3 magnesium, bio-identical progesterone as outlined.

Leanne wrote back:

So far so good… I started my progesterone cream 3 weeks ago and I feel great…

Of course am doing the I-3-C, kelp, B5 and Daily Essentials and magnesium as well.

I asked if she would send me a testimonial and here it is.

Progesterone cream saved my life and my job! I am in my peri-menopause and for several months (18) have experienced extreme issues with my period – I have missed 7 days of work in 6 months due to: HUGE blood clots so large I could feel them passing, blood gushing so extreme I could not leave the house for two and three days at a time, and cramps day and night impacting my rest. I just kept thinking this must be the last period… once I was forced out of my denial I contacted Brenda and her team – right away she recommended a daily regime which I started immediately because my purchase showed up on my doorstep the very next day. The results were that my very next period was "normal". I didn't realize how lousy I was feeling until I felt better. My aches and pains have also decreased dramatically. If you have any of these issues – don't wait like I did - contact Brenda and her team for YOUR personal needs! With Overwhelming Gratitude.

– Leanne T, Vancouver, BC

---

8 LIFESTYLE STRATEGIES
FOR A LIFETIME

If you wish to gain control over your health and your hormones, you must master the 8 **Lifestyle Strategies for a Lifetime** in the following chapters 15 to 22.

Although all of these strategies are important to restoring hormonal balance, I have tried to list them in order of priority.

CHAPTER 15

Lifestyle Strategy One: Drink Pure Water

B elieve it or not, water is THE most essential nutrient your body requires to function. You can live about five weeks without food but only five days without water.

Water plays many significant roles in your body. Everyone needs between 2 ½ (85 ounces) and 4 ¼ litres (144 ounces) of water every day (more if you are active, exercising or in a warmer climate).

Water is essential to life in many ways. You use water for every single one of your bodily functions, including digestion of food, absorption of nutrients, blood circulation and the removal of toxins and waste.

If you are not drinking enough quality water daily, you may notice fatigue, headaches, a lack of mental clarity and focus, difficulty losing weight and inappropriate hunger.

But in relationship to your hormones, the two key points you need to remember are:

1. Water is the main component of your blood and is needed to transport oxygen, nutrients, and <u>hormones</u> to your cells for use.

2. If your body does not get enough water, it siphons what it needs from the colon. The result is dehydrated stool, which is so sticky and gluey, it cannot easily pass from the bowel. Without adequate water intake you will have difficulty achieving and maintaining proper bowel function.

You must maintain proper bowel function so there is no buildup of toxic waste in the colon to burden the liver, as it is the liver that will break down excess estrogen and dump it into your colon for elimination.

Solutions

Aim for ½ oz of pure water per pound of body weight daily.

Pure water and non-caffeinated herbal teas are the only beverages that count toward your water quota. When you ingest caffeine and alcohol, you will have to consume above and beyond your daily requirement of water because metabolism of these beverages results in a 10-fold increase in your normal water loss through urine. This leads to dehydration.

Sip your water throughout the day or drink an 8 oz glass every hour. Do what works best for you, but don't wait until you are thirsty to drink your water; by then you are already dehydrated.

Pure Water

To obtain pure water economically, I highly recommend a solid carbon block home filter system, which will remove chlorine, bacteria, metals and chemicals. Filtered water can be put into reusable glass or stainless steel water bottles for convenience. Avoid plastic water bottles. Our environment can do without the plastic bottles and you can do without the chemicals that leach into the water. The longer the water sits in that plastic bottle, the higher the levels of chemical accumulation (especially if you tend to reuse plastic water bottles as they become weaker with age). When plastic water bottles are exposed to heat, they release even more chemicals, such as when you leave them in your car so you 'always have some handy'. Refer to **Lifestyle Strategy Five: Reduce Your Exposure to Xenoestrogens** for more details on how chemicals affect your hormones.

CHAPTER 16

Lifestyle Strategy Two:
Create Sugar-Free Days

The white crystalline substance we know of as sugar is an unnatural substance produced by industrial processes (mostly from sugar cane or sugar beets). It is refined down to pure sucrose after stripping away all the vitamins, minerals, proteins, enzymes and other beneficial nutrients. In this state, it is highly addictive and highly destructive.

The average North American consumes around 125 pounds of sugar each year. This is no surprise when you consider sugar is in everything from ketchup to salad dressing and canned soup to deli meat. Many of the foods you likely consume every day are packed with sugar. Food marketers are great at incorporating sugar into many products under a variety of aliases. Common names for sugar can include sucrose, fructose, dextrose, and high-fructose corn syrup – none of which actually sound like the word "sugar," but essentially mean the same thing.

Please don't fall for the hype stating AGAVE is a safe alternative. It isn't! Agave is very high in fructose *(anywhere from 55-80%, some even higher)* and is highly processed.

With the amount of sugar in our diets, it's no wonder we are seeing a continual rise in serious illnesses such as: weak immune system, diabetes, depression and/or mood swings, weight gain, heart disease, and cancer.

Sugar is EVIL but the three main concerns I have with sugar and your hormones are the following:

a. Nutrient Deficiencies

In Chapter 3: **Do We Really Need Vitamins?**, I explained that a food is either giving you nutrients or it is depleting your limited supply. If you are eating foods containing any form of added sugar, you are depleting your supply of nutrients. You cannot hope to <u>ever</u> achieve optimal health if you keep depleting the very nutrients you need for every function in your body including hormone production, adrenal function, proper bowel function and liver function.

b. Candida Overgrowth

In Chapter 9: **Fast Track Solution Four - Eliminate Candida Overgrowth**, you learned about the tenacious and toxic problem of a Candida yeast overgrowth. The first step in preventing and reducing the hold it has on your gut is to stop feeding it! Candida feasts on sugar.

c. Adrenal Exhaustion

In Chapter 10: **Fast Track Solution Five - Restore Adrenal Balance**, you learned about the importance of optimal adrenal function for hormone balance.

I explained the four sources of stress – emotional, physical, chemical and nutritional. You may not be able to control the emotional stressors in your life, but you <u>do</u> have control over the nutritional stressors, and sugar is a big one.

Every time you eat sugar, you are causing HUGE stress to your adrenal glands.

Regulating your body's reaction to sugar is one of your adrenal glands most important jobs. Every time there is a surge of sugar from eating sweets or refined starches (or both! Danish anyone?), your adrenal glands respond by sending out insulin to retrieve all of the excess blood sugar and store it as fat.

If your adrenal glands overreact and signal your pancreas to release more than adequate amounts of insulin, too much sugar is removed from your blood, which results in a low blood sugar situation. The adrenal glands then react to this new emergency situation by pulling sugar out of storage to restore normal blood sugar levels.

Sugar is a huge nutritional stress to your adrenal glands.

Solutions

Create Four to Five Sugar-Free Days Per Week

The easiest way to accomplish this is to choose one day a week and for the entire 24 hours do not eat any refined sugar. Then create two sugar-free days per week and so forth. Your goal would be to create four to five sugar-free days per week.

When I say sugar-free days, I am referring to refined sugar such as alcohol, ice cream, cookies, cakes, candy, chocolate and pop (and do not replace sugar with artificial sweetener which is extremely toxic). When I say sugar-free days, I am not referring to the naturally occurring sugar found in vegetables, whole grains, nuts, seeds and whole fruit (notice I said whole fruit as I don't agree with drinking fruit juice).

Go For the Gusto

If you are up for the challenge, try eliminating sugar entirely for a period of time, usually two weeks is best, and notice how you feel. You should experience higher energy levels, better moods, less food cravings, improved sleep and possibly some weight loss. You should also notice how much better foods taste and you shouldn't have as much of a sweet tooth.

Once you learn to eat foods without sugar, you will see why you don't need them in your diet and it will be a breeze to maintain a minimum of four to five sugar-free days per week.

CHAPTER 17

Lifestyle Strategy Three:
Eat Two Cups of Vegetables Daily

This strategy will go a long way toward helping your bowel function properly.

Fiber sweeps your intestines like a broom, decreasing the time it takes for the food you eat to pass through your intestinal tubing and be eliminated in a bowel movement. The less time food sits in your colon, the less time it has to rot, decay and produce toxins. Fiber can also absorb toxins, which helps eliminate them from your body.

Dietary fiber absorbs water in the intestines to provide bulk and soften the stools, so you can pass them quickly and easily without straining.

You need at least 25 to 35 grams of fiber daily to maintain colon health. The average North American consumes an average of less than 12 grams of fiber per day.

Vegetables will help increase your nutrient intake by not only providing more nutrients in their natural form, but by replacing or displacing foods that rob you of precious nutrients. For example, if you're used to filling up on pasta and meat sauce, try substituting it with two cups of veggies and meat and add the pasta (which is stripped of all nutrients) as a condiment, rather than the main component of the meal.

You may encounter advertisements which try to convince you their capsules or juice can replace your vegetables. Don't believe it. These well-marketed products might provide some of the nutrients found in vegetables and whole foods, but you can never duplicate Mother Nature, nor can you achieve your fiber quota with these types of products.

Solutions

To increase the fiber in your diet, start by eating two cups of vegetables every day (not including your intake of lettuce, peas, corn, mushrooms and/or potatoes). You can eat them – they just don't count towards your two cups. Certified organic vegetables contain more available nutrients and are free of toxic chemicals and genetically modified organisms.

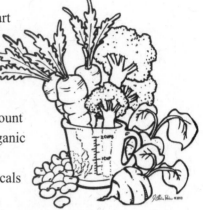

- *Lettuce* is a zero food, mostly water, low fiber and loaded with chemicals to keep it from wilting. If you eat lettuce, the greener the better (such as Romaine).

- *Corn* is a grain, not a vegetable. It is also a highly toxic food source now because at least 86% of all crops are genetically modified.

- *Potatoes* aren't bad vegetables; however they are so big and bulky, it would be easy to eat two cups of them, leaving no room for the healthy range of colored vegetables I want you to choose from, like leafy greens, broccoli, carrots, squash, beets, cauliflower and turnip, to name a few.

- *Mushrooms* I count as a fungus not a vegetable.

- *Peas*, unless you chew exceptionally well, you will spot them when stool-watching the day after you eat them or (if you aren't eliminating properly) maybe a few days after you have eaten them.

Legumes (i.e. lentils, kidney, and garbanzo beans) are good sources of fiber and protein, but wait until you have become accustomed to eating more vegetables before gradually adding beans. Incorporate them into your diet over several months. The digestive tract will adjust slowly and life will be far less gassy.

CHAPTER 18

Lifestyle Strategy Four:
Do Not Eat
Non-Fermented Soy Foods

S oy food has become big business. In a 2011 worldwide study, Global Industry Analysts forecasted the global market for soy foods would reach US$42.3 billion by the year 2015.

US-based soy grower Archer Daniels Midland (ADM) alone operates more than 240 processing plants and 330 crop-sourcing facilities in more than 60 countries on six continents.

The company recorded net sales of US$62 billion in the financial year ended June 30, 2010 and is also featured in the Fortune 500 list at number 39, right after Microsoft.

I am explaining this first so you understand why you are bombarded with so many reports on the health benefits of soy. However, I believe modern day soy and soy products are NOT health foods.

It is difficult to find the statistical proof for you because, as you can see, there are huge profits to be made by having the general public believe soy is a health food. Conversely, if there is no profit in proving otherwise, who is going to fund these costly studies?

I have done some digging and can provide the following facts for you. I hope after reading this chapter, not only will you decide against nonfermented soy food, but you will tell others as well. It is especially important to warn mothers that soy infant formulas put the baby's health at risk. The estrogens in soy can irreversibly harm the baby's sexual development and reproductive health.

THE MANY ISSUES WITH SOY

Writings about the soybean date back to 3000 BC. It was listed as one of the five sacred crops because it regenerated the soil for future crops. But it was the root, not the bean, that was considered beneficial. Ancient texts suggest the Chinese recognized soybeans were not fit for human consumption.

In their natural form, soybeans contain phytochemicals (phyto meaning from plants) such as phytates, goitrogens, and enzyme inhibitors that protect the soybean from the sun's radiation, bacterial, viral or fungal invasion and from being eaten by animals. But these phytochemicals have toxic effects on the human body.

Let's take a closer look at the issues related to eating soy food.

A. Soybeans contain high levels of phytates

All legumes contain phytates (also known as phytic acid) to some extent, but the soybean has one of the highest phytate levels of any grain or legume studied to date. Phytates are a substance that can block the absorption of essential minerals – calcium, magnesium, copper, iron and especially zinc – in the intestinal tract.

For most legumes, soaking is enough to break down most of the phytate content. However the soybean requires a long period of fermentation to reduce its phytate content to the point where it becomes fit for consumption.

This means fermented soy foods like natto, miso and tempeh have the lowest levels of phytate and are the best choices for anyone wishing to eat soybean products.

B. Soy contains high content of enzyme inhibitors

Your pancreas should produce digestive enzymes that allow you to break down your food and absorb your nutrients. Eating soy foods can impair this process because there are enzyme inhibitors in whole soybeans and unfermented soy products that are not completely deactivated during ordinary cooking.

The result can be gastric distress such as abdominal pain, gas, bloating and/or nutrient deficiencies, particularly in the amino acids that come from protein. Amino acids are the building blocks that make up all cells, hormones, and neurotransmitters (brain messages) in the body.

C. Soy contains goitrogens

Soy is promoted to women as being a great "hormone balancing food." However, soy is the exact opposite; it is an un-balancer of hormones! Typically, women adding soy to their diet will experience new symptoms or a worsening of existing symptoms of low thyroid function: irritability, fatigue, difficulty concentrating, depression, fluid retention, and headaches.

This is because there are substances in soy known as goitrogens, which can contribute to low functioning thyroid issues, because they inhibit the ability of the thyroid gland to make its necessary hormones. Also phytic acid blocks the absorption of zinc, which is needed for thyroid hormone formation.

D. Isoflavones, double-edged sword

Isoflavones are compounds found in soy foods. They are referred to as phytoestrogens (phyto means from plants) because their chemical structure resembles estrogen.

Depending on the type of estrogen receptor on the cells, isoflavones may reduce or stimulate the activity of estrogen. Isoflavones can compete with estrogen for the same receptor sites thereby decreasing the health risks of excess estrogen. They can also increase the estrogen activity adding to all of the health risks and symptoms of estrogen dominance I have brought to your attention.

Which way will it work in your body? Will it have a positive effect or a negative effect?

In case you still want to take a chance with the potential benefits of isoflavones, you should know that in 1997, researchers from the U.S. Food ánd Drug Administration's National Center for Toxicological Research discovered isoflavones are the goitrogenic compounds in soy foods which contribute to the depression of thyroid function.

So again, any possible benefits to consuming soy isoflavones are going to be negated by their anti-thyroid effect.

E. Soybeans are genetically modified

At least 85% of soybeans produced in the U.S. are from Genetically Modified (GM) seeds. Gathering evidence against GM foods is not so easy because there are billions of dollars being made on Genetically Modified products.

Note: Genetically Modified food has been altered at a genetic level to produce a better tasting, longer lasting, or more resistant product.

One of the reasons soy has been genetically modified is so it can withstand being sprayed with the toxic herbicide roundup. The weeds around the soy plant are killed off but not the soy itself, which makes spraying easy and supposedly increases profits for the producers of soy. Unfortunately the end result is you, the consumer, get a product which is contaminated with a deadly poison.

Thankfully the proof is starting to emerge. Just as I was putting together the finishing touches of this book, a study was published in the peer-reviewed journal *Food and Chemical Toxicology*. It found that rats fed a genetically engineered corn for two years developed massive mammary tumors, kidney and liver damage, along with other serious health problems. The corn chosen to feed to the rats is actually prevalent in the U.S. food supply. Even though this study is specifically on corn, I believe it clearly shows the toxicity of GM food.

Another study showed that hamsters fed GM soy were unable to have offspring and suffered a high mortality rate.

Despite evidence to the contrary, the U.S. and Canadian governments continue to maintain that genetically engineered crops are safe, resist disease better, and can provide much-needed food in starving nations.

When I am asked, "Are there really any benefits to soy?" The answer is, "Not as far as I can see."

Solutions

If you truly want to consume soy, the following list will help you minimize the dangers.

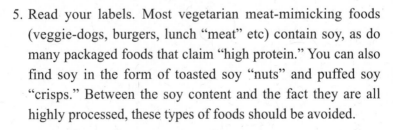

1. Limit your risks by not consuming it every day.

2. When possible, buy certified organic.

3. Try to eat only the fermented soy products: tempeh, miso, and natto. Tofu is not fermented.

4. Make sure your soy sauce is certified organic and naturally fermented.

5. Read your labels. Most vegetarian meat-mimicking foods (veggie-dogs, burgers, lunch "meat" etc) contain soy, as do many packaged foods that claim "high protein." You can also find soy in the form of toasted soy "nuts" and puffed soy "crisps." Between the soy content and the fact they are all highly processed, these types of foods should be avoided.

6. Remember, even though it is marketed as such, soy milk is not a health food. A great non-dairy alternative would be unsweetened almond milk or unsweetened hemp milk.

7. Do not eat edamame beans. Although they look and taste delicious, they are actually a young soybean.

CHAPTER 19

Lifestyle Strategy Five:
Reduce Your Exposure
to Xenoestrogens

Xeno means foreign, so xenoestrogens means foreign estrogens. This refers to environmental compounds that generally have very potent estrogen-like activity within your body, but they aren't real estrogens.

These xenoestrogens come from pesticides, herbicides, and fungicides, car exhaust, solvents and adhesives such as those found in nail polish, paint remover, and glues, emulsifiers, and waxes found in soaps and cosmetics. Nearly all plastics and dry cleaning chemicals are sources of xenoestrogens. And this is the short list.

Xenoestrogens can cause estrogen dominance which directly contributes to or will exacerbate ALL symptoms associated with menstruating and perimenopause.

I am sure you would agree that we are assaulted with chemicals and toxins in our environment. But you can't live in a plastic bubble, because even the plastic will give off xenoestrogens! You can't control air pollution, but you can significantly reduce your xenoestrogen exposure by controlling the **pollution in your own home and what you put on your body**.

WHAT YOU ABSORB

Most people don't realize just how much the skin absorbs and how efficiently these molecules travel through your body. If you are skeptical, then ask yourself how estrogen or nicotine patches work.

Still not convinced? Try crushing a clove of garlic and putting it between your toes and see how many minutes it takes before you can taste the garlic in your mouth. If you do this experiment, no further explanation is necessary.

You must be vigilant over the products you put on your skin because it absorbs everything.

Solutions

Here is a list of the personal skin care products you will want to replace.

- Toothpaste
- Mouthwash
- Shampoo and conditioner
- Soaps
- Body lotions
- Perfume
- Face cleanser, conditioner, toner and moisturizing cream
- Hairspray or styling gel
- Deodorant
- Make up
- Sunscreen

For a list of recommended non-toxic personal care products visit www.HormoneRollerCoaster.com

Two of the Worst Offenders

Even some of the most informed in the field of nutrition aren't aware of the linens and clothing factor. You are in contact with your sheets for approximately eight hours a day and in contact with clothing the rest of the time. This means what you wash and dry your sheets and clothing in is equally as important as what you apply to your skin.

Not only do these products contain xenoestrogens, but according to the Allergy and Environmental Health Association, both liquid and dryer sheet fabric softeners are "the most toxic product produced for daily household use." Most of the popular brands of fabric softeners contain many neurotoxins (substances that are toxic to the brain and nervous system) and other types of toxins.

Solutions

Replace your laundry detergent, fabric softeners and fabric softener sheets with non-toxic counterparts.

For a fabric softener, try adding ½ cup of baking soda to the water in your washing machine and let it dissolve prior to adding your clothes. Baking soda acts as a water softener and helps makes clothes super soft.

You can purchase or build a wooden drying rack and hang up some of your clothes to dry.

Have you ever smelled the freshness of laundry that was hung up to dry outside? This is how my grandmother used to do it and I just loved smelling the outdoor freshness. Sadly, most people don't have the space or time to hang up laundry any more. Also, of course, some cities are so polluted it might make laundry more toxic than fresh.

To give your laundry a nice natural scent, you can add a few drops of essential oils to your rinse water (I know, not the easiest thing to remember).

To prevent static cling, remove your laundry from the dryer before it's fully dry. Hang clothing on hangers to air dry the rest of the way and lay towels over the drying rack.

Beware of Plastics

Plastics are on the top of the list of what to avoid if you want to reduce your exposure to xenoestrogens.

Solutions

1. Never reheat or cook with plastic dishes or plastic wrap (one of the worst sources of xenoestrogens) in the microwave. If you are going to use a microwave (not recommended) it is much safer to use tempered glass or Corning Ware, etc.

YES — Metal Bottles **NO** — Plastic Bottles

2. Don't use bottled water. Buy stainless steel or BPA-free water bottles and put your own filtered water in the bottle to take with you.

What You Breathe In

Here is a list of household products you will want to change.

- Paraffin candles (alternatives can be beeswax candles or soy wax candles)
- Tub & tile cleaner
- Toilet bowl cleaner
- Window cleaner
- Room deodorizers (get rid of these altogether)
- Dishwasher detergent
- Dish soap and hand soaps (especially antibacterial ones)

Solutions

Review the commercial products in your home. At your local grocery store, you'll find there's a natural alternative for just about everything on the market. And they are usually quite cost-effective, as natural products tend to be far more concentrated so you use much less.

To freshen the air, place cinnamon sticks, nutmeg, whole cloves and sliced citrus fruit in a small pot of water on the stove. Bring to a boil and let simmer. The scent will be amazing.

To make a homemade air freshener try adding a few drops of essential oils in filtered water in a spray bottle.

Annie B. Bond is a renowned expert in non-toxic and green living. She recommends making a great all-purpose window cleaner by combining $1/4$ cup vinegar, $1/2$ teaspoon liquid soap or detergent (natural of course), and two cups of water in a spray bottle. Shake to blend and spray on your windows.

Go to www.care2.com for more of Annie's suggestions.

Search the Internet for natural alternatives to any product you wish to replace. You will be astounded at the number of options you have. Of course some work better than others. But with natural alternatives, there is no harm in trying them out.

The Food You Eat

Unfortunately, these xenoestrogens are everywhere. Commercially raised cattle and poultry are fed estrogen-like hormones as well as growth hormones that are passed onto humans when consumed. One half of all antibiotics in the United States are used in livestock. These antibiotics are a major contributor to hormone disruptor exposure. Feeds contain a myriad of hormone-disrupting toxins including pesticides, antibiotics and drugs to combat diseases in the animals. Much of this feed contains GM corn and soy.

Solutions

Whenever possible, purchase certified organic or at least hormone-free and antibiotic-free meats and poultry. Wild game is also a good choice. If your meat is not organic, trim fat from meat and skin from poultry and fish as that is where the toxins collect. Opt for wild fish, salmon especially, as farmed salmon will be fed pellets of fish meal with antibiotics and synthetic additives to obtain the pink color for which the wild fish are known.

Fruits and Vegetables

Approximately five billion pounds of pesticides, herbicides, and fungicides are used on our commercially grown fruits and vegetables every year.

I cross-checked many references and *The Shopper's Guide to Pesticides in Produce* (http://www.ewg.org/foodnews/) appear to have the most reliable list of the "dirty dozen" – the most highly contaminated foods and the lowest in pesticides.

<u>Solutions</u>

When buying produce from the "highest in pesticides" list, buy organic. If you can't, then peel the fruit or vegetable. If you can't peel them, then wash them well with diluted vinegar. This will help to reduce pesticides on the surface. Needless to say, this will not help to get rid of the pesticides inside. Discard the outer leaves of leafy vegetables.

SUMMARY

This is a very long list of things to consider changing to reduce your xenoestrogen exposure. My advice is to start with the two changes below and over time gradually make more changes.

Remember... progress, not perfection!

1. What you put on your skin (personal care and laundry products).
2. Do your best to make your house a plastic-free environment, starting with eliminating the use of plastic in the microwave and for your drinking water.

CHAPTER 20

Lifestyle Strategy Six:
Reduce Caffeine Consumption

If you have exhausted adrenal glands, caffeine will feel like it gives you a boost – and it does! It whips the adrenal glands into action and gives you a lift, followed by a crash, which means more wear and tear on your adrenals. If you keep this cycle going, eventually a hit of caffeine will no longer give you a boost. Would you whip an exhausted horse until it dies? I don't think so. You would be wise and give the horse as much rest and nutrition needed to recuperate. Please do the same for your adrenals.

It can be very challenging to control the emotional stress in your life, but you <u>do</u> have control over the amount of sugar and caffeine you consume. And trust me on this – caffeine and sugar are your two worst adrenal enemies.

If you keep overstressing your adrenal glands by kicking them with caffeine, you will continue to wear them down and you will either carry on feeling poorly, or you will need to be on adrenal support supplements for the rest of your life!

<u>Solutions</u>

Don't panic. I'm not suggesting you quit caffeine cold turkey, I am not even suggesting you quit caffeine. Here is what I am proposing:

If you have mild adrenal fatigue, reduce your caffeinated coffee consumption to a maximum of 16 oz per day

If you have moderate adrenal fatigue, slowly reduce your consumption to no more than 8 oz of caffeinated coffee per day.

If you suffer with severe adrenal exhaustion, you must cut out caffeinated coffee entirely until you can honestly say you are now rating yourself as having mild adrenal fatigue.

If you drink a lot of caffeine, then slowly reduce the amount, otherwise you will feel much worse before you feel better.

If you start to feel anxious at the mere <u>thought</u> of quitting caffeine, then you absolutely need to reduce your caffeine consumption.

*The more resistance
the more the need!*

What About Decaffeinated Coffee?

Methylene chloride is the solvent for the extraction of caffeine and it is an acknowledged animal carcinogen linked to liver and lung cancers.

<u>Solutions</u>

Please purchase organic coffee that has been decaffeinated by the Swiss water process.

Because coffee will make you acidic whether it is decaffeinated or not, you should still limit your intake to no more than 16 oz per day.

The body has an acid-alkaline ratio called the pH. It is measured on a scale of 0 to 14 – the lower the pH the more acidic your body, and the higher the pH the more alkaline your body.

Your pH balance has a profound effect on your breathing, circulation, digestion, elimination, immune defense and hormone production. Therefore, reducing your coffee intake can improve your pH balance, which in turn can improve your hormone balance.

What About Black Tea?

Black tea contains less caffeine than coffee but it also makes you acidic, so it is best to limit your intake to 16 oz per day.

<u>Solutions</u>

Green and non-caffeine herbal teas are fine to drink daily.

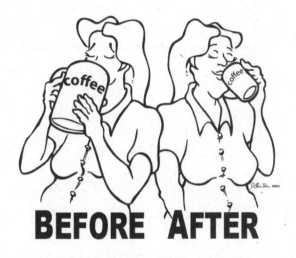

What About Other Caffeinated Beverages and Food?

Please be aware that caffeine can be found in many other foods and beverages such as green tea, energy drinks, sodas, chocolate, and even some supplements. No matter where you find it, too much caffeine is bad for your adrenal glands.

<u>Solutions</u>

Follow the recommendations in Chapter 15: **Lifestyle Strategy One - Drink Pure Water**. Adequate water intake should quench your thirst so you won't be as tempted to drink caffeinated beverages.

Follow the recommendations in Chapter 16: **Lifestyle Strategy Two - Create Sugar-Free Days**. This will help you dramatically reduce your intake of soda and energy drinks.

"Health is a state of
complete physical, mental
and social well-being,
and not merely the absence
of disease or infirmity."

~World Health Organization

CHAPTER 21

Lifestyle Strategy Seven:
Stop Drinking Milk

You have likely been brainwashed to believe that calcium is your saving grace for strong bones. Everywhere you turn you hear "drink your milk, eat dairy products, get your calcium," and when you think you have enough, the media keeps telling you to get more calcium.

What I am about to tell you may come as a complete SHOCK. I don't believe you should load up on calcium; in fact, I think the opposite. The more calcium you ingest, the more health issues you are going to have, especially when it comes to your hormones. **The only possible exception is if you take a calcium supplement that is properly balanced with magnesium and other nutrients, which help the calcium be absorbed and placed where it belongs.

I highly recommend you immediately stop drinking milk and severely reduce your intake of dairy products overall. This will not cause osteoporosis; in fact, it could literally save you from developing osteoporosis.

I have written an article about calcium and bone loss. For your free report "Important Facts That Can Make or 'Break' Your Bones" go to www.HormoneRollerCoaster.com

There are many reasons I suggest you stop drinking milk and drastically reduce your dairy consumption. One of the most significant factors is this:

Milk has a ratio of about eight calcium to one magnesium. The high calcium intake can cause a magnesium deficiency.

Remember:

(a) You can't make ANY hormones without an adequate supply of magnesium.

(b) Magnesium acts like a spark plug for the adrenal glands and for the energy system of every cell in the body.

(c) Magnesium works with vitamin B6 to reduce estrogen and increase progesterone, which of course helps you reduce your estrogen dominance.

(d) Calcium causes muscles to contract and magnesium causes them to release. Any constricted states in your body, such as menstrual cramps and headaches/migraines, will respond favorably to magnesium.

(e) Another contracted state relating to low levels of magnesium is improper elimination. Your body will try to eliminate excess estrogen through your bowels, but if your bowel does not empty properly, you will reabsorb the estrogen. This is another factor contributing to estrogen dominance.

<u>Solution</u>

My recommendation is to consume as little dairy as possible and eliminate milk entirely. Butter is okay, and eggs are poultry, not dairy. If you are looking for a milk replacement, you can use unsweetened almond milk or unsweetened hemp milk instead.

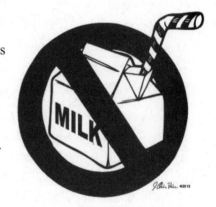

CHAPTER 22

Lifestyle Strategy Eight:
Eliminate Fluoride Sources

Fact: Fluoride has a negative impact on your total health BUT especially on the function of your thyroid

Fact: Up until the 1970s European doctors used fluoride as a thyroid suppressing medication for patients with hyperthyroidism (which is an over-active thyroid). Fluoride was utilized because it was found to be effective at **reducing** the activity of the thyroid gland – even at low doses.

Given the relationship between your thyroid and your hormones, protecting your thyroid from fluoride could dramatically improve your symptoms. The biggest threats come from fluoridated water and toothpaste.

Fact: There is enough fluoride in a half tube of candy-flavored toothpaste to kill a small child. In 2009, there were 24,547 calls to the U.S. Poison Control Centers due to ingestion of fluoride toothpaste (source http://www.fluoridealert.org). Check your toothpaste label. It says, "If you accidentally swallow more than used for brushing, seek professional assistance or contact a poison control center right away. As with other toothpastes, if irritation occurs discontinue use."

The membranes in your mouth are very permeable, so even if you use a small amount of toothpaste, rinse and spit, you will still absorb some fluoride in that 30 to 60 seconds it took to brush your teeth.

Of course, if you rinse well, then you are rinsing off the fluoride that is supposedly protecting your teeth, so why get fluoridated toothpaste in the first place?

Fact: Only 3% of Western Europe has fluoridated water. In Canada 40% of the water supply is fluoridated, and in the United States, about 60% of the total population gets their water from public systems that add fluoride.

Even if you don't drink the fluoridated water, you likely bathe or shower in it and the fluoride absorbs right into your body through your skin.

> *It is well documented that environmental contaminants such as fluorides are absorbed readily both through the skin and by inhalation ... Studies by Drs. H.S. Brown, D.R. Bishop and C.A. Rowan in the early 1980s demonstrated that an average of 64% of the total dose of waterborne contaminants, such as fluoride, are absorbed through the skin. (American Journal of Public Health 1984; 74: 479-84) —Fluoride: Drinking Ourselves to Death, Barry Groves, pp. 275-265*

Your food can be another potential source, depending on whether or not it has been made with fluoridated water. For example, where is your beer or wine made? Is it made in a city with fluoridated water? Instant powdered tea mix is exceptionally high in fluoride; now reconstitute it with fluoridated water and you have an even bigger dose of fluoride.

Solutions

1. Find out if your tap water is fluoridated or not. If it isn't, be very, very grateful. If it is, you have some decisions to make.

   Boiling will concentrate the fluoride rather than reduce it and freezing water is not helpful at all.

   Most filtration systems do <u>not</u> remove fluoride. They specifically avoid mentioning it in the advertisements because they <u>can't</u>

make claims about something they cannot do. Before you start looking for a trustworthy filter for your home, you need to decide whether you want one for your kitchen sink to filter the water you use for drinking and cooking or if you want a whole-house fluoride filter so you won't be absorbing the fluoride through your skin.

My next two solutions aren't very practical, but are worth considering.

2. You could lead or join the lobby in your community to reject the fluoridation program. Approximately 25 Canadian cities have rejected fluoridation programs and since 2010 it has been done in 64 North American communities.

3. You could also move to a city without fluoridated water.

4. Stop using fluoridated toothpaste. There are many natural brands available and you also have the option of brushing with silver solution gel.

Since I converted from fluoride toothpaste to brushing with silver solution gel, my gums and teeth are in better health. The most important part of dental hygiene is disrupting the bacteria that are responsible for dental plaque. If you let bacteria get between your gums and your teeth, it will attack your gums, penetrate the protective skin and invade tissues that attach teeth to bone, destroying this tissue and eventually attacking and destroying the bone itself. Silver solution gel eliminates bad bacteria. It is not only safe for brushing, but it is safe to swallow as well. For details on silver solution you can refer back to Chapter 9: **Fast Track Solution Four - Eliminate a Candida Overgrowth**.

"Each morning we are
born again. What we do
today is what matters most."

~Buddha

CHAPTER 23

Extra Support for
Painful Menstrual Cramps

The pain and intensity of menstrual cramps varies from woman to woman. Some women describe a dull ache or a feeling of pressure in the lower abdomen, while others experience such severe pain and pelvic discomfort they are unable to function.

Many women find the pain and associated symptoms so debilitating, they would rather have their uterus removed than go through the agony month after month. Even one of my teenage clients felt that way. This young woman missed school for several days each month because of the severity of her symptoms. She was literally begging her mom to allow her to have a hysterectomy.

Fortunately her mother convinced her to schedule an appointment with me first. After following my recommendations for only 30 days, the teen experienced such dramatic improvement that she stopped asking for a hysterectomy.

Not all women will get such quick and dramatic results, but with dedicated action, any woman can eliminate the pain or at least diminish it to a tolerable level within six months.

If you have skipped directly to this chapter, I assume you are in dire straits. If so, my recommendation is to get a medical checkup. It is important to know if you are dealing with endometriosis, fibroids, an infection, or cancer. Once you have a diagnosis, you can take appropriate action.

If you have an infection or cancer, you will want to seek out specialized treatment from your health care practitioner. You can approach either issue with traditional medicine, holistic medicine or a combination of both.

If there is nothing medically wrong (infection or cancer) or if the pain is from a fibroid or endometriosis, then I recommend starting at the beginning of this book and following the **Fast Track Solutions** and **Lifestyle Strategies For A Lifetime**. Once you reach this chapter, you should no longer have painful periods. If however the action steps have not provided enough relief, it simply means there is at least one **Fast Track Solution** or **Lifestyle Strategy For A Lifetime** you need to put more attention on. This chapter will help you define those areas. By closely following the guidelines, you can expect to become pain free!

THE ROOT OF THE PROBLEM

In general, women who experience intense menstrual cramps almost always have unusually high levels of prostaglandins.

Prostaglandins are chemicals produced by your body. One of their functions is to cause the uterus to contract every month and expel its unused endometrial lining in the process known as menstruation. However, if too many prostaglandins are produced, the uterus contracts too strongly and causes **painful cramps**. In fact, severe menstrual cramps are very similar to those a pregnant woman experiences when she is given prostaglandins as a medication to induce labor.

In the first half of your cycle, prostaglandins are low, then they rise sharply towards your period. The increase in prostaglandins is responsible for the variety of symptoms that can accompany menstrual pain such as nausea and/or vomiting, diarrhea, constipation, fainting, lightheadedness, dizziness, headaches and fatigue.

There are both 'good' and 'bad' prostaglandins. In the bad category is PGE2, a highly inflammatory substance that increases womb contractions and the sensitivity of your nerve endings to pain.

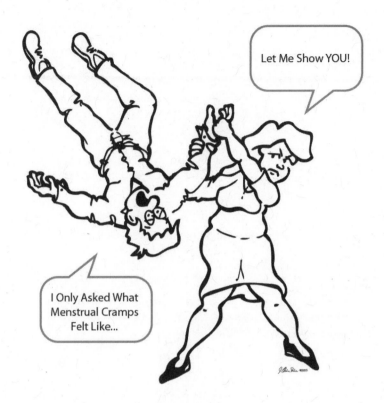

In the good category is PGE1. It prevents inflammation, as well as relaxes and widens blood vessels, which improves blood flow. Increased blood flow to the womb reduces pain.

Also in the good category is PGE3 because it helps to reduce inflammation and abnormal blood clotting. PGE3 blocks some of the inflammatory affects of PGE2 and can reduce arachidonic acid (AA) so your body can make more PGE1 (see chart 3).

The goal is to help the body produce "good" prostaglandins and reduce its production of "bad" prostaglandins.

Chart 3 on the next page shows the simplified version of how your body converts food components into different prostaglandins. If you understand the reasoning behind my advice, it will be easier for you to stick to my suggestions until you have reached your goal.

CHART 3

Omega 6

Linoleic Acid (LA) → found in Sunflower,
Sesame, Walnut, Flaxseed oil should convert to

Gamma-Linolenic Acid (GLA) → found in Borage,
Black Currant, Evening Primrose Oil should convert to

Dihomogammalinolenic Acid (DGLA)
will either convert to

PGE1 (the good   **OR**   Arachidonic Acid (AA)
anti-inflammatory,
anti-cramping prostaglandin)

PGE 2 (bad prostaglandin,
causes inflammation
and cramps)

Omega 3

LAlpha-linolenic acid (ALA) → found in cold water oily fish,
flaxseed and walnut oil should convert to

Eicosapentaenoic acid (EPA) → found only in
cold water oily fish can convert to either

Prostaglandin E3 series (PGE3)   **OR**   Decosahexaenoic acid
(DHA) → found only in
cold water oily fish

HOW TO REDUCE THE 'BAD' PROSTAGLANDINS AND INCREASE THE 'GOOD' PROSTAGLANDINS

Estrogen dominance is one cause of excess prostaglandins. Excess estrogen can over-stimulate the growth of the uterus's endometrial lining. The body then responds by increasing the production of prostaglandins in order to contract the uterus and push the excess endometrial tissue out during menstruation.

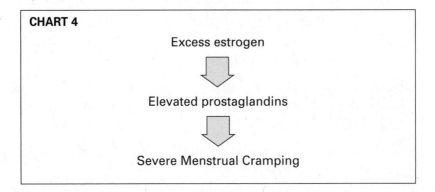

CHART 4

Excess estrogen

Elevated prostaglandins

Severe Menstrual Cramping

Part of the Plan

Every recommended action step in this book is designed to balance estrogen and progesterone, which should effectively stop your menstrual pain. If you currently have painful periods, do an honest review. What strategies have you been following and which ones did you skip or gloss over?

It is particularly important that you have been faithful to the **Fast Track Foundation** (Daily Essential Nutrients, B6 and magnesium citrate). All of the nutrients in the **Fast Track Foundation** are beneficial to balancing your hormones but there are some super stars in the group that will have a huge affect on diminishing your menstrual pain.

Nutrient Super Star Line Up

Vitamin B6, magnesium and zinc are at the top of the list of super stars. You need these nutrients in adequate dosages to make the good prostaglandins.

Also, **magnesium** acts as a muscle relaxant. Remember, calcium contracts and magnesium releases.

As reported by the *British Journal of Obstetrics and Gynecology* (2005;112:466–9) **vitamin E** is helpful for alleviating menstrual cramps and decreasing blood loss during menstruation. It helps to reduce production of bad prostaglandins.

Omega 3 fat from fish oil is extremely important in the treatment of painful periods because it gives you the EPA you need to make good prostaglandins (see chart 3).

Studies have shown women with low intakes of **omega 3** from fish oil have more painful periods than women who have a good intake.

A combination of **omega 3** from fish oil and vitamin B12 is more effective for relieving menstrual pain than just fish oil on its own.

Vitamin C has been shown to reduce inflammation.

Bioflavonoids are helpful with period pain because they help to relax smooth muscle and reduce inflammation.

Solution: Make sure you are faithfully taking the **Fast Track Foundation** as explained in chapters 5, 6, 7 and 8. It is important to take nutritional supplements for at least six months to ensure the nutrients required for the conversion are present in adequate levels.

Foods Can Increase Your Production of 'Bad' Prostaglandins

1. Too much omega 6 and not enough omega 3 increases PGE 2 (bad prostaglandins)

Both omega 6 and omega 3 fat need the same enzymes to complete the conversion to healthy prostaglandins. If you consume too much omega

6 fat there won't be enough enzymes for the omega 3 fats to make PGE3 (the good prostaglandins).

It is very easy to get too much omega 6 fatty acids from your diet because they come from vegetable oils such as corn, sunflower, safflower, soy, cottonseed and canola. These oils can also be hidden in snack foods, cookies, crackers and sweets. Omega 6 can also be found in nuts and seeds such as pistachios, almonds, sesame seeds, sunflower seeds, flax seeds, cashews, Brazil nuts, pine nuts, peanuts, pecans, pumpkin seeds, walnuts and hazelnuts.

On the other hand, it is hard to get enough omega 3 from your diet because it mainly comes from the fat of cold water fish such as salmon, sardines, herring, mackerel, black cod, and bluefish.

Solution: Cut down on omega 6 by reducing consumption of processed and fast foods. At home, use extra virgin olive oil for cooking and for salad dressings use either olive oil or cold pressed flaxseed or walnut oil. Walnuts and flaxseeds contain both omega 3 and omega 6 making them a better choice over the other vegetables oils which only contain omega 6.

Note: Do not rely on walnut and flaxseed oil to provide the omega 3 to make your good PGE3 prostaglandins. This is because the human body is not designed to convert the ALA (alpha-linolenic acid) from vegetarian sources to EPA in amounts sufficient enough to produce the desired effect (PGE3).

Eat more oily fish. And make sure you take your Daily Essential Nutrients as it contains omega 3 fish oil supplement.

Some women will get better results by adding a high dose omega 3 fish oil supplement containing a minimum of 660 mg of EPA and 330 mg of DHA to their Daily Essential Nutrients.

2. Foods high in arachidonic acid (AA) make more PGE2 (bad prostaglandins)

The main source of AA in the average diet is dairy products including milk, cheese, cottage cheese, yogurt and ice cream.

Solution: This is a good time to review Chapter 21: **Lifestyle Strategy Seven - Stop Drinking Milk**, where you will find this quote, "There are many reasons I am suggesting you stop drinking milk and severely reduce your dairy consumption." Beyond the reasons provided in chapter 21, this chapter offers you another reason to minimize your dairy consumption and that is your menstrual pain. Most women find their menstrual pain motivates them to try this solution, but if you are still struggling to give up milk and reduce the intake of your other dairy products, the second-best solution is to at least follow this advice for the two weeks leading up to your period.

3. Caffeine increases the output of prostaglandin PGE2

Solution: Please review Chapter 20: **Lifestyle Strategy Six - Reduce Caffeine Consumption**

Other Lifestyle Strategies Can Help Relieve Menstrual Pain

1. Healthy functioning adrenal glands can block some of the release of the inflammatory prostaglandin PGE 2

Solution: Please review action steps in Chapter 10: **Fast Track Solution Five-Restore Adrenal Balance**.

2. Sugar contributes to high blood sugar levels and the release of large amounts of insulin, which can trigger inflammation.

Solution: Review Chapter 16: **Lifestyle Strategy Two - Create Sugar-Free Days**. If you have not been able to be consistent with creating sugar-free days, then focus on the five to seven days leading up to your period and make those days completely sugar-free. Eating sugar may give you momentary gratification but days later will give you more menstrual pain.

I know pre-period can be the time frame you are most likely to crave sweets. But if you follow the **Fast Track Solutions** and **Lifestyle Strategies For A Lifetime**, your sugar cravings should disappear, or at least hugely diminish.

3. Dehydration aggravates menstrual cramps.

Solution: Review Chapter 15: **Lifestyle Strategy One - Drink Pure Water**.

If You Are Still Suffering

Following step-by-step, through the **Fast Track Solutions** and **Lifestyle Strategies For A Lifetime**, should have eliminated or at least reduced your pain considerably. If you are still seeking some relief, the next suggestions will be very helpful.

HERBAL SUPPORT

Wild yam is also considered to be a strong antispasmodic and is potentially anti-inflammatory. If you are already taking it for adrenal support, consider increasing your dosage from ovulation to period. If you aren't taking wild yam for adrenal support, then you can begin taking it from ovulation to period. You will have to experiment to find out the dosage that best suits you. Following are the maximum amounts I have suggested.

Based on the brand I recommend, which is 500 mg per capsule, you could take one to 2 capsules two times per day.

At the onset of cramps (should they still occur), you could take 2 capsules every hour until the cramping subsides.

You can read more about this herb in Chapter 10: **Fast Track Solution Five - Restore Adrenal Balance**.

Passionflower is known for its analgesic, sedative, and calming effects. It can also act like a muscle relaxant.

You will have to experiment to find out what dosage works best for you, but the range will be somewhere between 15 drops three times per day to a maximum of $1^{1}/_{2}$ teaspoons four times per day.

You can read more about this herb in Chapter 10: **Fast Track Solution Five - Restore Adrenal Balance**.

Red Raspberry leaves contain nutrients to tone and strengthen the uterine walls, making it a wonderful natural reliever of menstrual cramps. It can also help decrease a heavy flow.

It is important to realize the best results will be gained from consuming the herb on a regular basis. The dosage can be increased in the days leading up to your period. The longer you have been consuming the herb, the better your results. I would try it for a minimum of three cycles before deciding whether it is helping you.

It can be purchased in capsule form, as a tincture, or in dried bulk form.

Bulk: Steep at least one tablespoon of the dried herb in one cup of water for 15 to 30 minutes. You will need to drink three cups of tea per day.

Capsules: It will depend on the brand. Usually you would take a minimum of 1 capsule three times per day. Follow the recommendation on the label.

Tincture: Again it depends on the recommendation of the label, but generally you would take ½ teaspoon three times daily.

Non-herbal Support

Magnesium requirements tend to increase in the days preceding menstruation (as those of you with pre-period constipation and chocolate cravings can attest to) so I suggest increasing your dosage from ovulation to period. At the first sign of cramping, you can also take 2 to 3 capsules of magnesium and then 1 capsule every hour until cramping subsides, but be careful with your dosage as too much magnesium can cause diarrhea.

For a review on magnesium go to Chapter 7: **Fast Track Solution Two - Magnesium, The Miracle Mineral**

Natural Bio-Identical Progesterone Cream can reduce the output of PGE2. If you have not been using the cream, please review Chapter 14: **Fast Track Solution Nine - The Appropriate Use of Natural Bio-Identical Progesterone Cream** to see if it is suitable for you.

If you are already using natural bio-identical progesterone cream, you can increase your application to ½ teaspoon (approximately 40 mg of progesterone) twice daily during the week before your period. At the onset of menstrual cramps you can apply ¼ teaspoon (approximately 20 mg of progesterone) to your abdomen every hour till cramping subsides.

Please Note: I am not recommending natural bio-identical progesterone cream for the following women who are:

- under the age of 32
- taking Prometrium
- on any form of birth control pill
- on other forms of progestin (such as Mirena IUD)

Immediate Support

With perseverance, you will eliminate your menstrual pain. In the interim, here are some old-fashioned techniques you can use to ease your discomfort.

1. Castor oil on your abdomen may help. Purchase only certified organic premium quality castor oil. Take 30-60 minutes in the evening to use the castor oil on your abdomen. Either slather it on thick and cover lightly or make an actual pack with a piece of soaked flannel. For best results, do this for a couple of days before and during your cramping. Optionally, you can apply the castor oil or castor oil pack before going to bed, just be sure you lie on a towel and wear an old t-shirt so the oil doesn't mark your sheets.

2. A good old-fashioned hot water bottle on your abdomen can work wonders.

3. Soaking in a warm bath with Epsom salts is also helpful.

"Every human being
is the author of his own
health or disease."

~Buddha

You Have the Tools, But Will You Use Them?

This book was inspired and created through my desire for you to have the easiest, fastest and most inexpensive way to feel and look fabulous. I am so excited about the results that you will achieve, I can hardly contain myself.

I have done my part, and now it is your turn to do yours.

To help you on your way, I found a website (http://www.dumblittle man.com/2010/03/10-amazing-lessons-albert-einstein.html) that lists *10 Amazing Life Lessons You Can Learn From Albert Einstein*. I have quoted the two I believe can really assist you in reaching your health goals.

#1. *Don't Expect Different Results*

Insanity: doing the same thing over and over again and expecting different results.

You can't keep doing the same thing every day and expect different results. In other words, you can't keep doing the same workout routine and expect to look differently. In order for your life to change, you must change; to the degree that you change your actions and your thinking is to the degree that your life will change.

#2. *Perseverance is Priceless*

It's not that I'm so smart; it's just that I stay with problems longer.

Through perseverance the turtle reached the ark. Are you willing to persevere until you get to your intended destination? They say the entire value of the postage stamp consists in its ability to stick to something until it gets there. Be like the postage stamp; finish the race that you've started!

BRENDA'S 10 TOP TIPS ON
HOW TO FINISH THE RACE THAT YOU'VE STARTED

1. Start a health folder or health binder.

2. Go to the book section on my website and download all the free questionnaires, reports and checklists.

3. Fill out all the questionnaires right now so that you have a current list of all the symptoms that are keeping you from feeling your best. Now put those questionnaires at the back of your health folder or binder. Whenever you feel discouraged you can check the questionnaires to remind yourself of the progress you have made.

4. Buddy up with a friend who has also purchased this book. Set out your intentions and map out your action plan. Be accountable to yourself and to each other. Check in regularly to share ideas and your successes. Discuss any challenges you are facing and give each other feedback.

5. Read the articles on my website
www.HormoneRollerCoaster.com

6. Subscribe to my monthly newsletter on my website.

7. Attend one of my workshops or seminars. You will find event details on my website.

8. Join my Inner Circle Coaching Program. Details are on my website under "Support."

9. Contact me about speaking to your organization, corporation, church or charity event. Details are on my website under "Speaker."

10. Believe that your first responsibility is to your wellness. You can't do anything for anyone else, if you aren't well enough.

No matter what your age, you can have – and, in fact, deserve – quality of life: energy, mobility, radiance, focus, great moods, happiness and balanced hormones.

Yours in Total Health,

Brenda Eastwood